Never Skip A Beat

Thx for your Kind Words & support Linda xoxo

Linda Nowak

Never Skip A Beat

ISBN-13: 978-0-9988546-8-7
ISBN-10: 0-9988546-8-9

Published by: Celebrity Expert Author
http://celebrityexpertauthor.com

Canadian Address:
1108 - 1155 The High Street,
Coquitlam, BC, Canada
V3B.7W4
Phone: (604) 941-3041
Fax: (604) 944-7993
US Address:
1300 Boblett Street
Unit A-218
Blaine, WA 98230
Phone: (866) 492-6623
Fax: (250) 493-6603

I had the pleasure of meeting Linda at the Pacemaker Clinic in 2002. Over the years of following Linda at the Cardiac Device Clinic, I have seen her face and overcome much adversity. She has faced multiple surgeries and has unfortunately suffered from lead/device malfunction over her 40 plus year device history. Her strength, positivity and determination have carried her through the complex cardiac history that is hers alone. She possesses such a positive energy and beautiful smile. Even after receiving a shock for a life threatening heart rhythm while doing wind sprints at boot camp, she asks when she can get back to exercising. As well as being a wife and mother of two, Linda is a successful entrepreneur. Linda is a true inspiration on so many levels. It has been a pleasure to care for Linda over the years, and a privilege to call her a friend.

Sandra Dorey, B.N.
Nurse Clinician, Cardiac Device Clinic

Contents

Chapter One

"OUCH!" I YELLED. Everyone stopped and stared at me. I did not know what had happened.

I was in the middle of a high-intensity fitness class doing wind sprints and burpees when all of a sudden my pulse started racing. I stopped to get a drink of water, and it happened. I felt like someone had thrown a weight at my head.

The defibrillator in my chest had just shocked me. The employees called the paramedics because they had too. I did not want to go to emergency room because I was booked solid at my esthetics spa, but it's my heart we're dealing with, and I can't take chances. I'm shaken up, embarrassed, upset and most of all, yet again in my life, I'm reminded that I'm scared.

Fear. The emotion that dominated my life and that of my family since I was 12 years old when I got my first pacemaker, and it came back to the forefront of my awareness. I worked so hard to break through the terror barrier, but it was back, yet again.

At the emergency room in Lethbridge, I saw the cardiac specialist who I only see maybe once every five years because I always go to a specialist in Calgary. He asked me what I was doing when I got the shock and I told him I was doing Tabata, a form of high-intensity interval training. You go as hard as you can for 20 seconds and then rest for 10 seconds. You do this for eight cycles.

Well, he reminded me in a very stern manner that he felt the exercise was far too intense for my "condition.". He reminds me that I have an enlarged heart like it's the first time I am ever finding that out. "That's not enough recovery time," He says. "You should be doing an exercise like walking and never lifting anything heavier than 5 pounds." I didn't tell him that I usually squat over 100 pounds.

All those feelings that I worked so hard to overcome come rushing back. I'm different. I'm sick. Most of all, I'm afraid. I think to myself, "Maybe it is dangerous to exercise as hard as I do." Then I remember what life was like living in fear and I regain my composure.

I told the doctor that I wasn't feeling great that day. I was tired, a bit stressed, dehydrated and probably could have listened to my body a little more. We also have to consider the fact that I'm going through menopause as a contributing factor. He did not understand nor know the capabilities I have been able to push my body to…..the inner strength I possess.

I had broken through the terror barrier when I was 20 years old. I got my life back. I was living. I started feeling alive for the first time since I was 12 years old. Nothing was going to take that away from me again.

I decided that I was going to live my life and that my diagnosis was not going to own me. I made that committed decision when I was 20, and I have never looked back. Today I am in better shape than a lot of people with "normal" hearts. My doctors are so amazed by my health, given the complexity of my condition, I have been asked to partake in a medical study, which is currently being funded. They want to see if they can find out what I'm doing so they can use it to help other people with heart conditions.

This experience is the exact reason why I took this step to tell my story. Maybe you have just received a diagnosis, or you have been living with your condition for some time now. You may or may not have an ICD, but you are likely living your life in a way that is dictated by your condition. I'm here to tell you that you are not your condition and that you can choose to live the life you want to live.

I don't want you to be scared or overwhelmed by the activities that I participate in or the level to which I push myself physically. By no means do you have to do the things that I do. I can tell you that I did not start out doing what I do today. I did not even think it was possible. I took baby steps. I celebrated every small win, and I continued to work on myself every day. I kept my committed decision in the forefront of my mind, and every day it became more of a reality.

Since 2008, I have been blessed to be working with my specialist, Dr. Exner, a very forward-thinking man who can see me for who I am, beyond my cardiac condition. He is one of the very few people that I have encountered in the medical community who can work with me as a person with dreams and goals, rather than a patient with limitations due to a cardiac condition. Until I met Dr. Exner, medical professionals always had me focus on more negatives than positives. He is an example of the mindset that I believe more of our medical community needs to adopt o advance the health and recovery of cardiac patients and people with ICDs.

It is so critical to find the right support from your medical practitioners that I have included a chapter on building your relationship with your doctor in this book.

The device that I am fitted with is a defibrillator, and it will shock me if my heart becomes arrhythmic. Exercise and higher stress activity can put me at risk of arrhythmia and trigger my ICD. Now that I have been shocked twice, I understand the fear that people with ICDs have of being shocked. It also brings back the deep-seated fear that I have lived with my whole life. The fear that my heart will let me down and I will die. I have to remind myself of the conscious decision I made when I was 20 to live a full life.

Staying committed to my decision to live the life I want, the baby steps and celebrating the small wins has allowed me to live the life I do today. I can waterski, do high-intensity interval training, go boating and pretty much do anything I want. Small daily victories have amounted to such a big shift in my life that I often forget how far I've come.

I was invited to a medical event of approx 300 people with doctors, medical staff, and patients with ICDs, it was an event especially for individuals fitted with ICD devices. I was given the opportunity to speak with Dr. Stephen Sears at this event, and share my story of living with an ICD. His studies focus on this.

Once in the auditorium at the presentation, I could see that many in the audience were having trouble relating to being a person that could live a normal life, they did not see their device as a safety net as Dr. Sears stated. The questions that followed made it clear to me that people saw themselves as victims or possessed some special circumstance that did not allow them to live a normal life. I felt that people were not only medically, but mentally handicapped. My whole being felt so very sad at how absolutely crippled people were by this disease.

As I spoke to a few patients about my condition, they felt that I must not be nearly as bad as theirs. I think that they were thinking to themselves, "well I have this condition and, I can't do what she does." What amazed me most about the questions that were being asked, was how disabled people were by their conditions. One lady whose ejection fraction was significantly better than mine, basically meaning that her heart pumps more blood per heartbeat, told us how she was crippled in her house by her condition. Her days consisted of getting up for breakfast, going back to bed and watching TV, dragging herself to lunch exhausted and barely have any energy left to get through the rest of the day. I felt that this lady was not only physically limited but in reality, she indeed was mentally limited as well.

I felt so sorry for her that she is so handicapped by fear. She is not seeing her device for what it is. It's a safety net, that Dr. Sears spoke of, that it is there to protect you if you need it. No one Is safe from heart arrhythmias. I am a certified esthetician, and last week a 46-year-old woman, a customer at my spa dropped dead of a massive heart attack. She would have had a better chance of survival had she had my device. It's important to see how lucky you are to have this thing protecting your heart. Journalling helped me to see this for myself.

Most people living with ICD's are so fearful of the shock that they do nothing at all. The problem with the strategy is that the heart is a muscle and needs exercise. I always feared the shock, and I can tell you that now I understand and it is quite painful. I also know that when I was at my worst, I was in more pain doing nothing. Going outside and getting fresh air made me feel better. The more I did, the more I wanted to do. The better I ate, the more I wanted good food. I took baby steps and journaled about my small daily wins. I reminded myself constantly of all the things in life I am grateful for.

I understand that everybody's condition is different. Not everybody will want to do the same things that I do nor should they. But regardless of your condition, what you want and how you are progressing, your mindset is the most important key to living the life you want.

I was crippled by my condition for a lot of years. I went through being different in school, bullying and hating my life. My whole life didn't just change when I got the ICD. I have done a ton of personal development work and counselling for at least 15 years now. I believe in the power of positive thinking, and I know that is a huge key to my success.

I am what they call the question mark. My case is quite complicated. The doctors just could not figure out what was happening to me. I've had intensive surgeries including open-heart exploratory surgery. All they could say was that structurally, my heart was perfect, but electrically it was a mess.

When I was first diagnosed, I was constantly reminded that I was different. It was tough on my family, and I can only imagine how hard it was for my parents. My mom moved to Calgary to be with me for two months while I was in the hospital there. My two older brothers did not get as much attention as I did and I think that was hard on them as well.

My bedroom had to be put on the main floor because I could not climb the stairs, so I slept in the TV room. This meant that my brothers could not watch TV when they wanted to. My life became all about appointments. I had to go to the hospital two times a week to get tests done so they could send them to Calgary.

My whole life became about this condition. I'd hear my parents talking to their friends about their daughter with the pacemaker. I just wanted to scream "I'm Linda!" I did not want to be defined by this condition. But I guess this is normal for people with a serious diagnosis.

I get it. My parents were just following the doctor's orders, and they were afraid that I might die. But all that made it very hard for me to break out, stand up for myself and say, "let me try some things on my own!" Being a parent now, I can see how we protect our children. I cannot imagine this....when I asked my Mom how I handled everything; she replied that it was harder on them....I believe it!

It's easy to slip into being a diagnosis. I know. I've lived it.

It's OK to be where you are

Before a person is given a device, they have been sick for some time. The reason people get defibrillators is that they have dangerous heart rhythms. The device can give you freedom. You go from not being able to do activities due to bad cardiac rhythm to having the ability to participate in life again. The big problem is that most people don't get out of the sick mode. They stay focused on what they lack and what they cannot do. They don't appreciate the freedom that they have been given.

In most studies, Doctors state that their biggest obstacle they face with cardiac patients is getting people to motivate and challenge themselves. They said that with 80% of these patients, it was impossible even to get them to walk or take a gentle yoga class. They were not taking the required steps, and consequently, were not improving their conditions or quality of life.

So many people procrastinate in life. I think that this is the biggest reason that people with cardiac conditions and ICDs don't break through the terror barrier. You have to make the decision that you want to live your life and then follow through. Decide that there is nothing more important to you than getting to the point where you own your own life.

Do you want to know what my tiny steps to success are? I'll share them because these are what has allowed me to reclaim my life. For me, I wanted to learn how to break through the terror barrier and make decisions quickly. I had major anxiety due to my condition, probably because I thought of and feared death constantly. The fear is normal. When people get diagnosed with any disease, they are crippled by fear.

At one point in my life, I was given muscle relaxants to help control my anxiety, but they made me feel so awful, I did not like the controlling feeling that this medication had on me. I decided to work on my mindset instead. I did the serenity exercise, and it created a calmness of mind for me. In this exercise, you write out [something] for 90 days. While I was receiving some personal coaching, I was offered a serenity exercise that proved to be very helpful in calming the mind.

Any disease creates chaos of the mind. Imagine if you just got a diagnosis of stage four cancer. Immediately you think you're going to die. Calming the mind is critical to healing.

Get yourself a $0.33 notebook and write down all your small wins. Start meditating. The five minutes before you go to bed is so powerful. Instead of watching TV or surfing the Internet, do meditation or watch an inspirational, uplifting or funny video. I have included some of the favorite things I include in my bedtime ritual at the end of this chapter.

The most important thing for you is to get yourself to the point where you just can't take it anymore. To get to that point where you make the committed decision that you are taking your life back. Until you get there, your condition owns your life, not you.

It wasn't until I got older and moved out of my parent's house that things really started to change for me. The big turning point for me happened after I was married. I had an appointment in Calgary to change the settings on my pacemaker. My mom was still so involved in my life that she took me to the appointment, not my husband at the time. When we returned home to Lethbridge, the doctor's office called to tell us that they had gotten something wrong. They needed to get me back to correct it, but it was not urgent.

My mom woke me up at 4 AM and told me that we needed to get to Calgary right away. The whole way there I was in a mad panic, thinking that I was going to die. When I got there, they said, "oh you didn't need to come right away! We told you it wasn't urgent." I told my mom that she scared the living daylights out of me. At point I realized that I did not need someone else creating this much panic in my life. I was going to take charge of my own life. And from that point on, I began making my own decisions.

One of my girlfriends was an aerobics instructor so I asked her if I could just come and try one of her classes at my own pace. She told me it was absolutely no problem and that I could just do whatever I could and sit out the rest. I could not believe how great it made me feel. I felt so alive. I was so inspired that I decided to join aerobics training. I thought how cool would that be? Somebody with a pacemaker teaching aerobics.

I did get to a point where I taught a couple of classes. I didn't want to make a job of this. The main thing was that I didn't pass out and I didn't die. This was such an empowering moment for me, I had proven that I could do it and I haven't looked back.

I still have moments where I am crippled by fear today, but they don't last long. I have trained myself to search for the positive and to use the strategies that I know will get me back on track with my committed decision. My hope for you is that you will take simple steps to break through the fear and terror barrier. I am here to support you as you take baby steps and celebrate the small wins as you start living the life you want to live.

Bedtime Ritual

Watch short funny animal videos as I have a strong passion for animals, especially dogs

Read Something Positive

Deep breathing exercises

Ear buds in my ears listening to meditation.

Chapter 2

Linda's story...

Being diagnosed with a heart condition, suffering from heart failure or requiring a cardiac device can make you feel like life as you know it is over. It is a huge crippling problem, and the fear can be overwhelming.

I know because at the age of 12, I went from being a normal healthy kid who could play sports to a child with a heart paced at 72 bpm, who could no longer ride a bike or go swimming. Never in my life did I think that I would be crippled but from that day forward I lived most of my life in fear because I did not know what the heck happened to me.

If the 12-year-old me could have seen the me that I am today, my life would have been so different. I have learned valuable lessons in compassion, understanding, and perseverance. I would never trade the life that I had to go through to get here because I know that it was all necessary for me to enjoy all the things I have in my life today. Every one of us has a purpose on this earth. I believe my struggles has given my life purpose.

At 53, I am in better shape than most people in their 20s.

I train at a very high-level and I push my body and expect it to deliver. Most people I meet, or customers at my spa do not know that I have a device and my doctors just can't understand how I do all the things I do. I have a wonderful husband, two great adult children, a thriving esthetics spa where I work full time. Plus, I've recently started another pet waste removal business, which donates profits to the Local Animal Shelters and Humane Societies, as animals hold a special place in my heart. I do network marketing for a Company with Negative Ion Feminine Products, and a couple of other MSI's. I constantly keep creating ways of enriching my life and other lives around me, and on top of it all, I live the life I want to live.

Living this life became possible after I decided that I would no longer be a victim of my heart condition. When I broke through the fear and terror barrier, started trusting my body and decided that I wanted more from life, my life began to improve every day. The transformation is so dramatic that I often forget how it was to feel like I was crippled by my condition.

I know how terrifying it can be. Living in fear that any day might be your last. We place limitations on ourselves, hold ourselves back and do nothing in our lives to try and protect our precious life. But we have to see that at some point, this is not living. I was able to break free and I want the same for you. I know it may seem impossible, but trust me, you can do it. When people with cardiac conditions see me today, they think that my condition must not have been as bad as theirs, and that they can't do what I'm doing because I'm different.

I'm going to share my story with you now so that you can see that maybe my situation, although somewhat unique, may not be so different from yours. Most of us become our diagnosis and forget to be a person. This is not living. As you read my story, I want you to see where you are allowing fear and your condition to cripple you and how you can break through the terror barrier. Later on, I'll share exactly how I did it so that you can do it too.

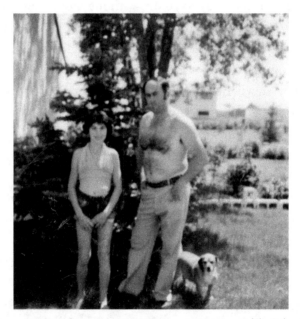

It was March 18, 1977. I was 12 years old. I had left school at lunchtime to walk up to the local candy store in town, I was with a friend, and passed out in an alley. When I came to, I was unaware of what had just happened. I got up and I went back to school. I came home with scrapes on my face from my fall and my mom asked me what happened. I told her that I had passed out but did not think anything of it. We had been out late the night before, and I did not get a good night's sleep.

It started to happen more often, and we became concerned. The doctor did tests and they thought I was hypoglycemic. After undergoing a glucose tolerance test it was determined I was indeed hypoglycemic and put on a strict diet. One Saturday, I was helping my Mom with household chores as we always got to go shopping after we were done. I was going to get ready to go out with my mom, and I passed out. My heart rate was dropping to 32 bpm. I was rushed to the hospital in Coaldale where they performed an ECG and found my heart rate to be dangerously low.

They transferred me by ambulance to the hospital in Lethbridge for monitoring; I was seen by the Cardiologist in Lethbridge and concerned with what was happening with my heart I was then transferred by ambulance to Calgary at 3 in the morning, where I met my first Cardiologist Specialist, Dr. Robert Sommerville. They did an angiogram, along with several tests and found no narrowing of arteries, and they determined I had to have Surgery. On April 7, 1977, they cut me open and broke my ribs to do open heart exploratory surgery. All they could determine was that my heart was good but the electrical part of it was not functioning properly. That's when they started calling me the question mark because to this day my condition is unknown. I was the guinea pig for several tests, but nothing was ever determined.

The procedure took nine hours, and they gave me my first pacemaker. Within 24 hours, my body was rejecting it. It had been placed in my abdomen and kept spasming in my system. It was a critical 48 hours, but it finally started to settle.

I was at the Holy Cross Hospital in Calgary for two months. My mom stayed with me the whole time, so they put her up in a room in the nurse's residence. My father traveled to Calgary on weekends to give my Mom a break; I still remember him traveling up in a record-breaking snowstorm in 1977, leaving my brothers behind with help from my Grandparents.

I had a chest tube that needed to be stripped of blood every 48 hours. My ribs were spread open, and there was massive scarring. It was a really hard and painful recovery.

I finally left the hospital just after the May long weekend. I now had a demand pacemaker in my body that was set to 72 bpm. It would kick in when I needed it whether I was sitting or walking. I was living within my limitations.

I had missed two months of middle school and was returning with only a month of school left. It was really hard. I remember sitting in class not knowing what was going on. I was a straight-A student before I went into the hospital. Math was especially difficult, and I had no idea what the teacher was talking about. I was frustrated and struggling.

I was not allowed to do gym class, and I could not play any contact sports. The device was the size of a cigarette pack, and I had to wear loose clothing to accommodate it. I could no longer play volleyball and baseball or any other sports.

The biggest frustration was that my mind kept saying I can do this but my heart and my body would not let me do anything because I would feel faint or pass out.

The school year ended, and I spent the summer adjusting to my new condition. In the fall I started grade 8, and that's when things got really rough. The bullying and teasing started.

When you can't partake, people look at you like you're different. I wanted to change schools. I wanted to go where no one knew what had happened to me so I could avoid the kids that bothered me. I would go over to my grandma's house to eat lunch because it was a safe-haven for me. I was always a very outgoing person but this experience was making me turn inward. I had become scared and fearful, but I tried to pretend like nothing bothered me. I really wanted to be cool, but I could not be. I just couldn't fit into the stylish clothes. Fortunately, I did have some great friends who stood by me. I have my bad moments and bouts of crying, but eventually, I adopted and accepted my life. However deep down, I just wanted my old life back. I was living the typical victim lifestyle and feeling sorry for myself.

Gym class got modified for me, and the teachers tried to include me by letting me keep score and other things that I could do. Sometimes the pacemaker would act up, and my parents would have to come and get me. I was always going in for monitoring and tests, like twice a week. It was never smooth sailing.

The kids would call me battery operated and pretend to short circuit when I walked past them. I was afraid to go to school; I felt ashamed of my condition.

I had a demand pacemaker, so my heart was not paced full-time however it was becoming dependent on it so I did not feel very good. I felt dizzy, and it seemed like my heart was just not keeping up with me. I felt like I was not getting enough juice in that 72 beats a minute. It just was not enough.

One day, it seemed like something just wasn't right. I told

my mom, and she took me to the hospital and asked them to monitor me for 24 hours. They said that there was nothing wrong but my mom said that I just kept complaining that I did not feel right. They found that the device was malfunctioning. If this had not been detected when it was, I would have died. They gave me another device and changed out the battery.

These devices were never supposed to fail, and now it had let me down. This just elevated the fear that I was living in.

In 1981, when I was 15 years old, I had another episode. I told my mom that I was not feeling well. They found that my pacemaker was malfunctioning and they rushed me to Calgary with a temporary pacemaker in my arm. They decided to install a full-time pacemaker.

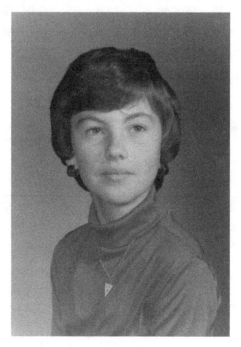

My limitations seemed to become more pronounced. An artificially paced heart does not contract the same way as a normal heart. Nobody could understand what was causing the deterioration in my heart function.

I tried to live like a normal teen, but every day, the chatter in the back of my head would remind me that I was different. I always thought that I would love to wake up one day and not have to think of my heart. I always had to wonder whether my heart was beating normally or not. Is today going to be a good day or bad day? I was always in fear of the bad days.

They told me that the device would never quit, but mine had. I had lost trust, and I was very fearful. At age 15, I was not feeling well. I knew in my mind that my heart was not functioning properly, My Mom took me into emergency and insisted they keep me overnight for monitoring. The next day in the afternoon my device had failed, and I had to have a temporary pacer placed through the vein in my arm to keep me alive to get to Calgary for surgery.

Everyone treated me like I was fragile and I was always being told what I couldn't do. My parents did what any good parent would do and tried to protect me. This was the best thing that they knew to do for me, and I know that they did it because they cared so much.

When you're different, and you feel like you're fragile, you just keep feeling like a victim. While I was living at home it never even occurred to me that I could get out of this victim mode.

Life changed once I moved out of my parent's house. Because nobody was watching over me, I could start to be myself a little more.

When I was 19 years old, and I had just finished high school, I got my dual chamber pacemaker in. This allows your heart to function more normally and I was the perfect candidate for it because I was young. It could go as low as 60 bpm and as high as 150 bpm at a topper rate. I remember the day when I woke up from the surgery, and they got me up to walk. My heart started to speed up, and I started to feel anxious because I was afraid of that feeling. They told me that I just experienced a normal heart again.

I had to adjust to my life again because now I had a fluctuating heart. Once I got used to it, it was wonderful. I felt like I got my life back. I started to become more active and began pushing my boundaries because that's just who I was.

I did things that I would never tell my mom about because I know she would just worry. I started to play baseball on the team, and that was awesome for me. I started waterskiing and spent my summers on Kootenay Lake. I became a lot more active and started to feel like a normal person again. I did have some setbacks from overdoing it, but it was all worth it.

I still had some limitations in the movement of my arms because I did not want to displace the lead wires or bump the device but that did not hold me back from trying new activities. My parents were always afraid of me doing too much because they were constantly thinking about the risk it posed to my health. My doctors were the same way. But I knew that I needed to try to do the things I wanted to do to be happy.

This device was reliable, and I had a long stretch without any episodes of malfunction. I just needed to get the battery changed every three years and then as the battery life improved, it went to 5 years.

In 2007 things changed again. I had my cleaning business at that time, and I was driving down the West Side Hill. I felt like I was going to pass out, so I called my husband. He came to get me and took me to the hospital. Nothing showed up, but I knew something was wrong. They thought it was just anxiety.

They would do threshold tests and bring my heart rate down to see how low it would go before I felt faint. This made me feel awful, and the whole experience was terrifying. The tests kept coming back normal, but I knew something was very wrong. I could tell my circulation was not good because I felt the tingling in my hands and feet. It was really frustrating.

Finally, after about two months and multiple tests including a thallium scan, an angiogram, heart ultrasound and a MUGA scan, they found the problem. The MUGA scan revealed that my heart ejection fraction, the amount of blood it pumps per beat, was in the low 30s. A normal ejection fraction should be around 60. This put me at extreme risk of sudden cardiac death as I was experiencing dangerous heart rhythm.

All the trust issues that I developed when I was 15 years old and my first device quit on me came rushing back. They did not believe me when I said there was something wrong but if I had been left at home, I could have potentially had life-threatening heart arrhythmias.

I was getting the same feeling I had back then, and the anxiety was overwhelming. This time, I met with over nine different doctors and specialists and none of them could come to any conclusion. Some tests came back normal which contradicted some that came back abnormal. I was afraid to be left alone. Once again, I was crippled by fear. I was scared to do anything because I felt like something really bad was going to happen.

I started having dangerous episodes, and fortunately, they were able to capture one of them when I was in the hospital. They were at a loss as to what to do.

A cardiac expert, Dr. Derek Exner, had taken on my case in 2007. He was the first doctor that I felt I could really work with as a real person rather than a case number and diagnosis. He truly appreciated my drive to push my limits and live a normal, fulfilling life. He suggested that when someone has been paced for so many years on the left side of the heart, it stops contracting properly. I fondly remember an appointment I had with my follow up nurse in Calgary and Dr. Exner popped in the room and spent close to an hour with my husband and myself taking a plastic mold model heart and explaining my heart's condition to us. Being a child when this all happened to me, I never received an explanation of my condition, just that I was considered a big question mark. It felt so reassuring to have someone to take the time and make sure I had my questions answered.

In 2008, while I was in surgery, Dr. Exner disagreed with the other specialist who was operating on me. This doctor wanted to replace my pacemaker with another CT Device but Dr. Exner had a different plan. He decided to add a third lead to my heart and put in an ICD Device instead. He proposed that this extra lead would help strengthen my heart and the defibrillator would be there as a protective mechanism against arrhythmia. Thanks to his certainty, he won the argument, and I am living with this setup today.

After the surgery, a couple of weeks had passed, and the incision site was causing me grief. I went to my local doctor and my found out my incision was at risk of infection, and I was put on three different rounds of antibiotics. It never seemed to clear up. Fortunately, my neighbor is an emergency doctor, and while talking to him in the yard one day, he discovered that I had a fistula.

I was taken to the hospital in Calgary because they were afraid that the infection would attach to a lead and go to the heart. It took three surgeries to get the infection under control. I had a lot of wire in my system, and they were trying to extract it. Unfortunately, the first surgery had dislodged my lead wires for my new device, the surgery and recovery were over nine hours. There had been a lot of damage to my chest and shoulder region, and it was causing a great deal of pain. I had a fourth surgery. Upon completion of my final surgery just before I was discharged from the hospital on the final checkup rounds, they discovered I had a collapsed lung and needed to have a chest tube put in. Once down in the OR Suite, they could not get a vein to put in anesthesia, so they just froze the sight and put the chest tube in my chest. I still remember the pain I went through, one nurse noted to my husband of my unbelievable strength. I was determined to leave the hospital after that as my daughter had a final piano recital. She was performing a song she wrote called "Night Sky," and I did not want to miss that performance for anything. Sure enough through my strong will and determination I made it to her performance chest tube in and all. I then went to emergency at our local hospital and was able to have the chest tube removed the following day.

I still remember the intense amount of pain in my upper body that I felt. I could not stand straight or sleep on my back. They wanted to send me to a pain clinic in Calgary, but I don't even like taking a Tylenol when I have a headache. There was no way I was going to start taking heavy duty narcotics.

I didn't work for over a year. I gave up my cleaning business and focused my energy on my healing. I did holistic body balance and acupuncture. It was crippling for some time, but I pulled out of it. I got back into the beauty industry because it is easier on the body. The nerve damage still affects feelings in my fingers and certain days I still feel a bit off, but I now focus my energy on how grateful I am to have pulled through it all.

I developed a more grateful attitude towards my life and my device. I slowly started incorporating activity back into my life. I started walking, then working out, and I got back to waterskiing. The more active I got, the better I felt.

I'm extremely active now. In my workouts, I have done high-intensity workouts including sled pushes, swing sledgehammers and tire flips. The only thing I don't do is chin ups because it puts stress on the leads. I also take care of our acreage.

Life is great now. No one would ever know I had heart issues by looking at me. I don't like people to know I'm different. Most people don't even know I have a device. I spent so much time trying not to be different that now I know it is possible to break through the fear and live a normal life.

To this day, I don't like going for tests. Threshold tests make my stomach turn, and the thought of surgery gives me anxiety. I still have some deep-rooted fears, but I also have strategies I can count on to get through to the other side of them and live my life.

It makes me really sad to see people who are living with cardiac issues so crippled by fear. I don't know each and every one of your cases, but I do know that you can break through the terror barrier. You just need to do something, anything and you will feel better.

I've shared my story so that hopefully you can see that I am not much different from you. I have improved my heart function just by being active. My last MUGA scan was between 45 and 46. I would not even qualify for an ICD with these numbers. Normal is around 60.

Dr. Exner applauds me for what I do and has taken a special interest in my case because of the freedom he feels it can bring to so many other cardiac patients. That's why I felt compelled to write this book.

If you are tired of being fragile and living your life in fear, you don't have to. I discovered the mindset necessary to break through the terror barrier and live a normal life despite your condition, diagnosis or device. In the chapters that follow, I will share exactly how I did it and what you can do to start living the life you want to live.

HEART FUND CANVAS

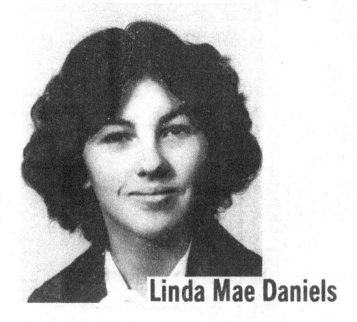

Linda Mae Daniels

The Heart Fund Canvas Kicks off Wednesday, February 7th...Linda Mae Daniels, age 14, is one the the many Alberta youngsters with a heart problem. She is the daughter of Mr. & Mrs. Herman Daniels, 4312-3 Ave. S. Two years ago she had corrective heart surgery & now is enjoying school activities & enjoys being outdoors, all with the help of a heart pacer. Thanks to medical research, Linda & others like her, can look forward to a normal and active life. Your donations makes Heart Reserach possible. The home to home canvas is scheduled for Monday, February 12th. Approximately 900 canvassers will blitz the city residents in aid of the fund. Lethbridge's share of the $1,000,000 goal for Alberta is $50,000.

BIG BOOST FOR HEART FUND CAMPAIGN

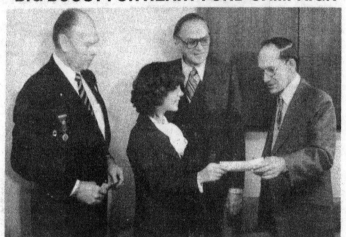

Photo by Terry Bland

. . . A total of $2500.00 was donated towards the Lethbridge branch of the Alberta Heart Foundation's campaign for $50,000.00 by two Lethbridge organizations at a Heart Fund luncheon recently. Shown above on the right is Robert Neville, secretary of the Loyal Order of Moose, as he hands a cheque for $1500.00 to Linda Mae Daniels, Miss Heart of Lethbridge. On the left is John Hargreaves, first vice-president of the General Stewart Branch of the Royal Canadian Legion as he waits to present to Miss Heart a cheque for $1,000.00. Watching the proceedings is Dr. John Callaghan, eminent heart surgeon of Edmonton, and honorary chairman of the Alberta Heart Foundation. Mr. Hargreaves is recovering from open heart surgery performed by Dr. Callaghan while Linda Mae Daniels underwent corrective heart surgery two years ago and is now enjoying a normal and active life. Linda Mae, aged 14, is a Grade 9 student at R. I. Baker School in Coaldale. She is the daughter of Mr. and Mrs. Herman Daniels of 4312 - 3rd Avenue South.

The business canvas for funds is now underway while the house-to-house canvas will start on Monday with approximately 800 canvassers blitzing city residents. The Alberta goal of the Heart Foundation is $1,000,000 for heart research.

Chapter 3

Getting Beyond Fear and Limitation

The hardest thing that cardiac specialists have to deal with among their patients are the fears and lack of motivation. According to Dr. Steven Sears, for the most part, the patient is their own biggest limitation.

I had the honor of meeting Dr. Sears and sharing my personal story at an event held in Calgary for people living with ICDs. Dr. Sears thought it would be inspiring for people to hear about someone who was living an active, normal life with an ICD. To my surprise, as I sat and listened, what I thought would be motivational had the opposite effect.

I had been enjoying living for so long that I had almost forgotten how crippling the fear surrounding my condition was. The saddest thing for me was the resignation and disbelief coming from the audience. Any suggestions about the possibilities that exist for them because of research, technology and their devices were met with opposition. We heard a lot of, "Yeah but I can't cause my condition is different." People got up and spoke about their limitations and focused on things they felt they lacked, like energy and strength. They were unaware of the safety net that Dr. Sears spoke of that they possessed to protect them.

Right away, I knew what the problem was but sadly, he did not get to shift the focus of the discussion. They saw their condition as the problem that was keeping them from a full life. I remember how life was when I thought that way. It wasn't pretty. I grew up with my condition and have been living with it for over 40 years. I either had to develop a different mindset towards it or live a miserable life.

Until I had attended that event, I had forgotten about the mindset that pervades heart patients and people with ICDs. Dr. Sears helped me to understand that my biggest challenge when addressing this audience about their possibilities is that I need to start at a kindergarten level. I like to jump out of the starting gate now but I realize that I wasn't always like that.

Dr. Sears has developed a model for people who want to live a full life with a heart condition. Based on all his research and case studies, he has come to the simple conclusion that all you need to do is keep calm and take a step forward. When we are consumed by fear, we aren't calm. We lack focus on what is good and what is working. We have all this chatter about what we can't do, and we don't see the possibilities.

I know how all-consuming a heart condition and living with a device can be. The doctors told me that my device would never quit on me. They said that Medtronic would be out of business if things like that happened. But when I was 15, I knew something was wrong with my pacemaker. I just did not feel right. They told me it was nothing but if I had not made a fuss about it, and my parents had not insisted they admit me overnight for monitoring I would be dead, as my device had quit the next day while in hospital. My parents did not even have the opportunity to come sign the proper paperwork for them to take me into surgery. I was rushed down to the surgical suite, and a temporary pacemaker was placed in my arm. Afterwards, I was transferred to Calgary Hospital.

Fear became my controlling paradigm. My doctors assured me that everything was okay but how could I believe them. How could I trust my device when I had already been let down?

I know what it is like to suffer from paralyzing anxiety. I was afraid to drive, I was terrified by the highway, and I always had to have someone with me in case something went wrong. My doctors wanted to medicate me, but I didn't want to be on any meds. I felt so trapped.

My condition had consumed my whole life. I did not do anything that put any demand on my heart, and I never put myself in any situation where I could not get help if something went wrong. I finally got so fed up with being crippled by my fear that I had to make a change. I could not live like this anymore. I needed to do something. Anything. But from my point of view, everything just seemed so risky. I mean I felt like my life was at stake!

I'd be lying if I told you that I no longer have any fear. I just deal with it a lot better now. I now know that the secret to overcoming fear lies in the power of the mind. I discovered that my limitations were not due to my condition but rather to the mindset about my condition. Now, whenever I feel the fear begin to surface, I do my best to get a hold of it right away.

Loosening the Grip of Fear

I wanted to do so many things that other people did for fun, but I felt like it was too dangerous for me. Anytime I even thought about doing something physically active; the anxiety would start to rise within me. Just thinking about attempting something new would cause physical symptoms in my body. I'd get short of breath, my heart would act up, and I'd feel exhausted. How could I even try to do something when thinking about it made me feel this bad?

I had heard that overcoming fear was a mental game, but I did not know what that meant exactly. I decided that I needed to radically change the way I thought, or I would be like this for the rest of my life, which was not an option. I felt so useless and incapable, and I wanted to feel like I could do something if I wanted to. I realized that I was always thinking about what I could not do and why I was not able to accomplish something. This made me feel frustrated, depressed and trapped. Whenever I thought about doing something new, these were the feelings that came up, and I would back down because of them. I built up a happy exterior to mask what was really going on inside.

When I asked myself why I wanted to try new things, something interesting happened. I got a stir of positive emotion in me. I realized that I wanted to feel a sense of accomplishment or even power. Most of all I wanted the freedom to be able to do things and live the life I wanted to live. These were the feelings that were missing in my life and living in fear was keeping me fixated on the negative emotions. I knew then that I needed to think in a way that made me feel positive and uplifted.

Get a Good Feeling First

I really wanted to get active and healthy, but I did not think I could. This made it impossible for me to be successful with any attempts. I knew I had to get a new perspective on physical activity so I asked myself why I wanted to do it in the first place. I wanted to feel strong, have energy and feel good. I wanted to be motivated and excited about being active. I wanted to feel the accomplishment of deciding what I wanted and getting it.

Again I found myself feeling energy stirring inside me. I decided that I needed to activate this energy, so I focused on it. I pictured myself in an aerobics class and being able to participate. I visualized what it was like to finish the class. I felt the excitement and energy inside, and I knew that I would be able to go to a class. I might not be able to do the whole thing or participate at a high level, but I was not feeling held back from going. I was still scared, but I was going to do it. I was always trying to push my limits to test how far I could actually go.

Let Go of Expectations

I wanted to go to my friend's aerobics class, but I was afraid of not being able to do it. My friend was so fit, and the other people in the class would be so much better than me. Thinking about these things made me feel like backing down and ultimately, a failure. I knew that if I was going to escape from the hold of my fear, I just had to go. I had to be okay with where I was at and whatever happened. I told myself that going to the class was my victory and it made me feel good.

I decided that I would simply set myself up at the back

of the class and do what I could as long as I felt good. I was not going to pay attention to what other people were doing. I was just going to focus on my participation and how good it was that I was there. I felt like I could do that and it felt good.

Take the First Step

Once you can think about what you want to do and you feel good, it's time to take the first step. Forcing action when you are feeling negative emotions is probably not going to get a good result. When you get a good feeling first, you set yourself up for success.

I advocate taking baby steps. You don't want to make a giant leap. It's not only likely to backfire; it's probably dangerous. Don't worry. There is plenty of time for the small actions to add up and become big changes. You just need to start where you are and give yourself a break. So what if you are not awesome right out of the starting gate. Just getting there could be your win for the day. Tomorrow you can take another step.

All Outcomes Are Good

Once I started believing that all outcomes are good, my whole life changed. I had been so used to focusing on what I did not achieve and what had not worked that I always seemed to get negative results. When I started looking for what was good and what had worked, I started finding goodness everywhere.

I was totally uncoordinated and lost the first time I tried aerobics. I modified everything, and sometimes all I could do was just step on and off the step that I had on the lowest possible level. I was out of breath, exhausted and I hurt for days after. Part of me was embarrassed and wanted to explain to the other people that I had a heart condition, but that was focussing on my limitations. I stayed through the whole class! That was a major victory for me. My friend that taught the class was where I chose to put my focus.

The next class I was not totally lost. I could feel the energy moving in my body, and I thought to myself, "I can do this!" I was getting the same feelings of accomplishment, upliftment, and power that I had wanted when I thought about why I wanted to be active in the first place.

Build Positive Momentum

Momentum happens when something gets set in motion and picks up speed like a snowball rolling down a hill. The same thing happens with our thoughts and emotions. The momentum of thought can work in either direction. We can have a downward spiral of thought or an upward one. The danger of leaving your thoughts unattended is that they tend to spiral downward.

It takes conscious practice to build positive momentum. The easiest way to do this is to always look for something to appreciate and to celebrate every little win. Keep taking the small steps forward and always acknowledge the good in any outcome. Soon you will find that you don't even see any negatives.

Exercise to Release Fear

In the chapters that follow, I will be guiding you through the steps to overcoming the limitations of your condition and living the life that you desire. The first thing we need to do is get a good feeling inside when we think about something that we don't have or aren't doing in our lives now because of our condition.

1. If you did not have the limitations of your condition right now, what would you do?

2. If you had no fear and you could not fail, how would you feel doing or having what you answered in question 1? (List the feelings. Do it in the 33 cent notebook I told you to get!)

3. What can you do in your life right now that makes you feel those feelings?

4. What could you do today to experience those feeling?

Don't worry if you don't know how to answer right now. Getting beyond fear and limitation takes focus and practice. In fact, the rest of this book is really just a guide to help you develop the skills you need to constantly overcome the obstacles and see the opportunities that are there to help you create the life you want despite your condition.

In the next chapter, you will discover the importance of meditation and how beneficial it is for people with heart conditions. For now, keep practicing finding a good feeling and focusing on the positive in every outcome.

Chapter 4

The importance of meditation

WHEN I FIRST got diagnosed with my condition at age 12, I was afraid. Very afraid. My mind was constantly filled with monkey chatter that drowned out any possibility of positive thoughts. I would wake up, take my pulse and wonder what was going to go wrong today because of my condition. My fears about my health, the bullying at school and what my life could look like dominated my focus. It was stressful, depressing and exhausting.

A 12-year-old is supposed to have fun and enjoy life, not worry about life or death. It was unbearable, and I needed to survive so as a natural defense mechanism, I distracted myself. I focused on things that made me feel joy and connection. I would play the organ and took regular lessons, or I would sing because I felt calm when engaged in music. My mind would quiet for the time I was doing it and I would feel more peaceful afterward. I would also be able to think more clearly.

Unconsciously, by wanting to escape the pain that my thoughts were causing me, I had discovered the benefits of meditation. I had found a way to quiet my mind and allow the negative momentum of my thoughts to slow down. The reprieve I got gave my mind a chance to see things with clarity for a bit before the monkey mind took over again and the stress and anxiety set in. Naturally, I found myself doing something to quiet my mind every day so that I could calm my mind and feel peace.

Of course, not many 12-year-olds practice meditation, and in the 1970s you were considered weird if you did but today it is a widely accepted practice for gaining control over your thoughts. My recent pursuit of personal development has led me to a daily practice of meditation and my research shows me that my escape into music gave me almost the same results.

Calming the mind will help you deal with your condition better and let your body heal. I know this through my own experience and my dad's as well. At 52, he was diagnosed with bladder cancer and given a survival expectancy of 30%. At that time he took the conventional medical route. His cancer came back in his mid 70's and he had to have a kidney removed. I said to him, "Dad, just let me take care of you. What's the use of getting upset? It just raises your blood pressure." I helped him through the practices I am sharing with you in this book. My father has always been a very spiritually connected man, with a strong belief in God. He was living in complete fear. Now he knows how to focus on what he wants. He's a completely different man. At 79, he can vacuum and make a pot roast, two things we would never have believed until we saw them.

Ultimately, my goal in meditating is to create a positive momentum of thought that is focused on what I want to see and experience in my life. So often, our train of thought is moving faster and faster in the negative direction. Before we can even start to experience positive thought momentum, we have to bring the train to a stop. Only then can we begin to build momentum in the opposite direction.

Meditation slows the momentum of thought. It gives your mind a reprieve from the monkey chatter and allows it to have glimpses of new insights. This allows you to see the same situation that you see day after day with fresh eyes. The potential opens up for you to seize an opportunity that you never noticed before and create a change that affects the course of the rest of your life. These opportunities exist all around us however we rarely act on them because we are so busy responding to the same things in the same old way. When we meditate, we break out of this pattern and begin to consciously build new ones. This is why meditation helps you to build the life you want.

Meditation has been integral to my own success at continually building a better life despite the limitations of my condition. None of my life achievements would have been possible if I did not meditate or quiet my mind. I would have stayed miserable, paralyzed by fear and watching my condition deteriorate. I probably would not be alive today. Everything you have read so far and all the strategies that I will share in this book have been and are greatly enhanced by meditation practice.

Meditation Can Be Easy

People often have strange notions of meditation involving candles, crazily twisted postures and weird chants. There certainly are practices that do involve those things, but you don't have to do any of that to meditate. It can be as simple as sitting undisturbed, with your eyes closed and focusing on your breath for fifteen minutes. All you want to achieve is a slowing down of your thoughts.

You may find this difficult to do because you find yourself thinking the whole time. I promise you that if you simply take the time to sit undisturbed for those fifteen minutes and you do it every day, you will get the benefits. By just carving out the time to meditate, you are committed to your well-being, and your intention alone will begin to influence your thoughts.

How to Start Your Practice

Find a Time that Works for You

The easiest way to get in the habit of meditating is to do it at the same time every day. You may choose to get up fifteen minutes earlier so that no one disturbs you or perhaps you want to do it right before bed.

Find a Comfortable Position to Be Still in

Ideally, you want to be comfortable and move as little as possible for the duration of your meditation. If you need to shift to get comfortable, that is okay. You can sit or lie down. Just be sure that if you are lying down, you don't fall asleep. You can sit on the floor on a cushion, but that can be tiring. You may prefer to sit in a chair or propped up in your bed with pillows. It doesn't matter. Start the habit and adapt your posture as you go. You can cover yourself with a blanket to make sure you stay warm.

Find Somewhere to Place Your Focus

To break away from the monkey chatter, it is necessary to get the mind to focus on something else. Your breath can be a very good place to keep your attention. Notice the flow of air going into your lungs and out. You'll start to observe the different qualities of your breath like the sound, feel, depth and speed. Observe and be curious and interested in your breath. Set a timer so that you know when to end the meditation.

Another strategy that I like to use is guided audio. I will often find a meditation on Youtube to listen to. You can find thousands of different guided meditations of all different lengths. Someone will guide you in keeping your focus on some intention. There are all kinds of meditations of varying qualities, so you just have to find one that you like. It is important to make sure that you like the background music (if there is any) and that you resonate with the person guiding it.

Here are a couple of meditations that I have found very powerful. They are guided audios for purchase. (I have no affiliation with the sellers)

https://sellfy.com/positivemagazine

http://www.cdbaby.com/Artist/ElaineMartin

The second meditation is specifically for children dealing with sickness and anxiety. It provides step by step guidance.

Notice Any New Thoughts or Insights

The purpose of meditation is not to stop the mind from thinking. All we want to do is to slow down thoughts so that we get the opportunity to gain insight or have new thoughts that we have not experienced before. When the monkey mind is going, it is impossible to hear anything but its incessant chatter. When we slow thoughts down, new thoughts get a chance to surface and be noticed.

A new thought or insight can lead to a new action or decision. It may seem insignificant at the time, but a small action can change the course of your life and lead to a massively different outcome.

The Benefits of Meditation

Many people feel a sense of calm when they meditate that lingers for a while after. The benefits of meditation can be subtle yet massive at the same time. Often we don't notice them because we are just going about our day and acting on our impulses. But as our impulses change, we start to get new results. New results start to spark new ideas and new actions. This creates momentum and cumulative change. After meditating for a while, people are often surprised to see that they have achieved goals that they have never been able to make headway on and let go of weights that they have been carrying for years.

Meditation is incredibly beneficial for heart patients and people with ICDs. That is why I created these meditations based on practices that I have found most transformative in my life for overcoming the obstacles and limitations due to my condition. Most of all, they have allowed me to break free of the fear that ruled my life and build the life of my dreams. I know you can do this too. All it takes is the commitment to wanting something different and dedicating fifteen short minutes a day to calming your mind.

Once you have a desire to be, do and have more in your life and it feels good to you, it's time to start understanding how to work around the limitations that you perceive about your condition. Meditation and a positive attitude are definitely the most important tools that you can use to create more in your life, but we do also have to respect the fact that heart conditions and ICDs do present some challenges that we must understand and learn to work with. In the next chapter, we will talk about getting the facts about your condition.

Chapter 5

Getting the Facts About Your Condition

GETTING DIAGNOSED WITH heart disease or any disease for that matter is life-changing. A doctor comes in and gives you the details of what has happened, and you're left there wondering what this means about you and your life. You may think things like, "Why me? What did I do to deserve this? There must be some mistake! My life is over."

Maybe you were living a healthy lifestyle and did everything right. Maybe you were doing everything wrong and just waiting for this to happen. Or perhaps it just hit you right out of the blue. However it came upon you, things have changed, and you are no longer the same person you were before the diagnosis. You have to accept that things are different and that you will need to take a different approach to living your life than you have up to this point.

You get faced with limitations that you have to accept and learn to live with. Maybe you can't climb a flight of stairs. This can trigger fear and depression and the feeling that you'll never be the same again. If this is left unchecked, it develops into something even worse than the actual condition. It's called "victim mode," and it WILL ruin your life.

The first thing that attacks you is the fear. Fear of the unknown. When you have a heart condition, you become intimately involved with fear, and you better learn how to work with it and master it, or it will run your life. I know because fear pokes its head into my life on a regular basis and I have had all sorts of relationships with it.

The fear of the unknown can be crippling. For me it was, "Am I going to live or die?" I was a child when I got my diagnosis so I did not have any concept of what I could have done to deserve this. I just knew that I was normal and then I was not normal. I was limited, and I wished that I could just be normal again.

I was always wondering what my future would look like, what my life expectancy would be and whether I would be able to have children. Everything got more difficult. Travel was a problem, especially going to the United States and needing insurance. It's hard to get coverage with a heart condition.

There are two major factors at play here.

1. There is the actual diagnosis of the condition
2. There is your perception of yourself

It is very important to realize the difference between these two things if you want to master the fear and live the life you want to live on your terms. When you can see that the diagnosis is just a set of facts and parameter that you have to work with, with the right perception, it is possible to create anything you want. When you understand that the perception you have of yourself is the only thing that you can change in the moment, you have power.

You can look for the different events throughout your life that led to the deterioration of your health, but this is only going to feed the problem. Asking yourself why this is happening even if you think you did everything right will just feed the fire. There is a multitude of emotions that flood your mind and body after the diagnosis, but the fear of the unknown is the most crippling thing.

Your routine gets totally disrupted, and you're left wondering how your lifestyle is going to change. You find yourself asking what your future will look like and whether you will ever be the same again. You're always questioning whether you can eat something or not, if something you do will be harmful to the condition or if you will die. It is very easy to live your whole life stuck in this cycle of fear and doubt. It's when you learn how to see beyond the fear and make conscious choices despite it that life starts to become something amazing.

Because this happened to me when I was 12, I didn't have all the learned fears that we get as adults. I only knew that my parents and teachers were freaked out, but I wanted to play and be normal. I just did what kids do, and I pushed the limits. If my parents and doctors said don't do something, it made me want to see what I could get away with. I found out that there were a lot of grey areas. After all, I was just a kid trying to have fun.

This evolved into a whole life of experimenting and pushing the limits. I developed the mindset that I would not let this define me. I wanted to feel as normal as possible, and I would seek out help and find whatever options and modifications that would allow me to do this. As I got to understand my body and my device better, I learned to work with how far I could push things, and I discovered that once I was beyond the fear and doubt, that it was a lot farther than I ever thought.

Doctors will always tell you the limitations of your condition and what you can't do. That is their job, and it is how they are trained. You won't ever hear them telling you to experiment with your condition and move beyond your limitations. This is a huge disservice in my opinion because it keeps you focused on the fear and doubt and it just grows until it becomes absolutely crippling. But you can gain control of these negative emotions and begin to fill your experience with positive and good feeling emotions if you are willing to commit to choices that empower you. You must decide to seek out help and start taking actions that make you feel as normal as possible. I did it despite the complexity of my condition and against the recommendations of my doctors and my parents. It has allowed me to do things that no one ever thought would be possible and I continue to be able to do more new and amazing things in my life.

It's a cycle that you learn to master. The fear and doubt never goes away, and your condition has its ups and down. We have no control over what is happening in the moment, but we do have control over what we choose to focus on. I know it can sound like a broken record. People always say that it's not what happens that matters. It's the choices you make, what you focus on and the actions you decide to take in the moment that make all the difference. When you have a heart condition with or without a device, it becomes absolutely imperative to grasp this and live it if you want to enjoy a great life.

I still get pulled into fear and doubt from time to time because of circumstances that arise due to my condition and the device. I view myself as having a safety net device in me that protects me from heart arrhythmias, which can be fatal in even the most seemingly healthy individuals. I see it as a special advantage that I have over everyone else. However, since I received a shock from the defibrillator in it, I have some limitations right now. I can't go to the gym and do interval training until they figure out what tripped the device and I go three months without another episode. The limiting belief of, "here we go again," pops up and rears its ugly head and I can flounder in the uncertainty but I know I have power over my perception. So until I get the okay to go back, I am going for walks and doing yoga.

Normal people don't have to think this way. They are not faced with the circumstances that a heart condition can present. There is no monkey chatter of "what will the doctor say? Or will this cause a heart attack?" But I also know that by gaining mastery over my perception of my condition, I have gained superpowers in every part of my life. Normal people don't do this either. But you can!

The majority of people with heart conditions are so worried about their condition acting up or their device going off that they won't even take a little step forward. One guy said he was afraid to work on his car because he thought it would throw off the timing of his device. I've changed the spark plugs and oil in my car without even thinking twice, but

I realize that I've had a lifetime of exploring my limits and expanding them.

I understand why it can feel like your life is over. It was absolutely devastating for me to go from being a normal kid one day to being different and not allowed to be a kid anymore. All I wanted to do was play but I couldn't because I was told that everything could harm me. I did not understand what was going on or why this had happened to me. None of the doctors did either. My memories of life before the disease are almost like a dream. It doesn't even seem real to me anymore.

Getting diagnosed later in life can make it a lot harder to separate the two factors. Your condition and your perception of yourself all become muddled together. More of your life was spent in your pre-disease, "normal" condition and your memories are of what life was like without the limitations. Nobody likes to be told that they can't do something by someone else. But as adults, we have learned the rules. We listen to doctors, and we defer to their recommendations.

While I did not recognize it at the time, I was fortunate not to have had to deal with my diagnosis with an adult mind. I had the child mentality of, "why no?" and the negotiating tactics of a child that does not understand "no." I would keep asking until I got my way. If they said I could not do one thing, I would ask if I could do something else. Most of the time I would just keep rephrasing the question until they were so sick of me asking that they said "yes."

Now I do understand and work within the realm of the physical limitations of my condition and my device. I don't want to provoke a shock, and I certainly don't want to die. When I see people on Facebook doing crazy things like jumping into ice water for fun, I know that it would just be suicide for me. Extreme body temperature changes would change my heart rate too rapidly, trigger my device and too many things could go wrong. I know my body, and I weigh the risks and rewards. Feeling invigorated by an ice bath is not worth the jolt I would get from my defibrillator.

I have never tried bungee jumping and have been told not to, but I can understand why this would not work with my particular condition. My daughter wants to go skydiving, and I was told absolutely not. These things disappoint me. Maybe the average heart patient would not think of doing these things, but I do. I think of how I could do things in a way that works within the parameters imposed by my condition. There's always a way, and if you're determined, you'll find it. I did win on water skiing after all!

I have always wanted to do a fitness competition, but the diet and training is way too strenuous on the body and heart in particular. There are enough cases of seemingly healthy athletes dropping dead training for them. As an esthetician, I have clients that are training for competitions, and I wax the athletes before the competitions. I can now see just how strenuous it is and don't have the desire to put myself through that.

That being said, I have definitely trained intensively with goals and eaten on nutrition plans that have gotten me in exceptional shape. I also have the pictures to prove it. My goals have evolved and, I work out because I enjoy it, not because I have something to prove. I am my ideal weight and people always comment on how well I take care of myself.

I do it because I love to. Not because I have to due to my condition.

When you are living every day like it could be life or death, it can actually be quite fulfilling. You start to see that there are no coincidences and that you really do attract what you need, when you need it. But you need to have the right headspace and perspective of yourself to see it. My biggest stroke of "luck" was to get Dr. Derek Exner as my heart specialist. He was exactly the type of doctor that I needed to support me in pushing my limits. Having this relationship with my specialist has been so pivotal in my life and lifestyle that I have dedicated a chapter to developing a relationship with your specialists.

When I spoke to him about my goals and desires, he did not shut them down. Instead, he encouraged me to be creative and play within them. I felt like I was supported and safe in my experimentation without the fear of being reckless. Most heart specialists are disappointed that their patients are not more active and are not interested in physical activity. The don't realize that they are a big part of the problem when they shoot down everything that a person wants to do. Derek Exner's approach to living with a heart condition with or without a device needs to become the norm among heart specialists.

I didn't just jump from passing out every time my heart went above 72 bpm right into high-intensity training when I got my dual chamber pacemaker. I asked my girlfriend who was teaching aerobics if I could try her class. I wanted to set myself up at the back so that if I felt it was too strenuous, I could leave the class. Well, I made it through and found out that I liked it. I went again and was able to do more. The more I went, the better I felt.

You can simply start wherever you are. There are many more beginner options now than back in the 80s when I got into fitness. Most gyms offer classes tailored towards people with health conditions or seniors and the instructors are trained to modify the exercises to suit a person's ability. There is also a great variety of different kinds of classes. Find one that interests you and tell the instructor that you are a heart patient. You will be pleasantly surprised by how accommodating they are.

Just start by accepting where you are today. Don't compare yourself to the pre-diagnosis version you remember from a long time ago. When you can simply do what you can do now, you start to see what is possible. And the more you show up, the more you find yourself trying new things. This is how you find out what your possibilities are.

I started very gently, making sure that I did not do anything that would hurt me. First I experimented with aerobics, and I found out that I was not as fragile as I was led to believe. I moved on to weight training. When light weights got too easy, I experimented with medium weights. This opened the door to a whole new realm of possibilities for my body and what I thought was possible. As my perception of myself changed, surprisingly, how my body responded to my condition changed as well. Medium weights became easy, and I tried heavier weights and that is how I got to where I am today.

When my condition is in an area of uncertainty, I do yoga because it has wonderful benefits for my body. I feel like my body needs this because as an esthetician I am often bent over and working in strenuous positions. I take my walks because it feels good to be outside and I take care of the work that needs to be done around our acreage.

When I started water skiing, I had to be very careful that I did not bang the device. As a woman, my bathing suit had padding in the cup which provided an area where I could make sure the device was protected. I bought a really good life vest that provided an added layer of padding over the device. Whenever there was an obstacle, I just kept asking Dr. Exner what I could do until I found a solution. I always wanted to do more and just kept taking baby steps. And my health continued to improve.

Start by expressing to your doctor that you want to do more. Most doctors want their heart patients to be active anyway. Never go out and start doing vigorous exercise without consulting with them. Just do a little bit and start learning how your body responds. As you listen to your body, you will get a clearer understanding of your condition than any doctor could ever have. This has saved my life on numerous occasions.

If you feel like this is a really big step, that's okay. Most people feel like a victim of their condition at first. I know because I was there. I can also tell you that it does not have to be crippling and you don't have to stay there. I still have my moments, but now I know that I need to take care of my mindset first. When my body is being affected by my condition, and I am getting frustrated, I know that it can be a slippery slope. If I don't take control of my perception of myself, I fall into the victim mentality and get crippled with fear too. But as soon as I find myself there, I use all my tricks to get back in control of my mindset.

When would I see people doing things that I want to do but can't I used to get really angry. Now I focus on things that I can do. It's really is mind over matter. If you think you can't, you are probably correct. You cannot see the possibilities without putting in some effort. Remember, it only needs to be a baby step, but that little movement forward will show you the next step. You may feel like everything good was stripped from you, but I assure you, there is still so much good inside you. Once you start playing with possibilities you will see it, and you will want to see more.

I have always been telling Dr. Exner what I want to do and I see that I can have it. My experience with most people with heart conditions is that they want a better life, but they don't think they can have it. It takes constant focus, but it is not hard work. We just need little wins every day. It's keeping the focus and mastering the perspective of yourself that is the hard work. But it does not need to be hard, and I will share some simple methods I used to gain it.

When circumstances arise in my condition, and I need to refocus, I always go back to the basics that I am sharing here. The first time my defibrillator shocked me, I was doing wind sprints and burpees. That should not normally have tripped it, but I was tired and dehydrated that day. That may be the reason. The second time, I was not pushing myself to the same limit. I was only doing a warm up. Dr. Exner was as surprised as I was. Now I am going to Calgary for a battery of tests. They are looking for a focus point and if there is the possibility of doing ablations, but first a change in meds is the first step.

The fear of the unknown is upon me again, and it is kind of crippling. Why did it happen if the doctor wasn't expecting it? Why am I getting these shocks? Is this going to change the course of my life again? Now I'm nervous to elevate my heart rate and have been doing very limited activity. I know I'm overthinking it and when you start overthinking things, it creates that panic in your life.

I have recently been contacted about being a potential candidate for a study; it's about how heart patients and people with devices can live healthier more active lives. I do things beyond anything they have ever seen, and they want to know if this is possible for others. I'm not special, and I know that, but I also know why most people don't do what I do. The heart patients at the lecture Dr. Sears was giving were asking questions that were loaded with fear. They don't know that the fear is running their lives, not the condition.

Some of their questions are so ridiculous in my mind today, but I have had those thoughts. I know that in their minds these are real things even though they are just thoughts. They have it rooted in their minds that their lives are over. This is simply not true, and I will show you how to overcome this.

All you have to do is think of things that make you happy. Use your imagination. Read and put yourself in a good mindset. Go to a funny movie or watch a comedy on Netflix. Laughing is by far the most healing medicine on this planet. Find people who are fun to be around and appreciate how much better you feel by spending time with them. Some people are always looking on the bright side of life. Only hang out with positive, fun people who lift you up and make you feel good about life.

Once I was old enough to move out of my house, I realized that I was absorbing stress from my parents. My mom recently said that she thought that the disease was harder on them than it was on me. She was right. Their perspective of me was not what I saw, but their influence over me had an impact on how much I did. It was not until I was on my own, making my own choices that I began to discover how much power I had over my condition.

Get away from the support groups. They are negative are filled with information about what you can't do and what you can't have. They are never focused on uplifting thoughts or possibilities. Avoid anything that makes you feel worse about yourself or your condition. Getting your mind in the right frame is the most important.

How do you move away from a negative mindset? Replace the fear with laughter. That is the key to getting moving. Keep calm and look for the funny things in life. Meditate, go for a massage, sit in a bubble bath and watch funny animal videos. It is simple to start there.

If you are reading this book, you ready to get better. You are searching for steps, and it is time to take the first one. Do something different or new. Something out of your usual routine. It does not have to be big, but it will break your focus from the fear. Everyone fears the shock, and I truly understand the fear because it is painful. I feel like a dog with an invisible fence right now.

Start creating a calmer mind by making yourself laugh. Those little things start getting you into a better mindset. When your mind becomes calm your body relaxes. To get a strong body, you need a strong mind. Every athlete knows this.

Tell yourself that you are going to pull yourself out of this. Decide that you want to start vibrating higher levels of thought. You will feel the vibration in your body, just like the good feeling you get when you are laughing with someone you love. It's the constant work to keep the vibration up, but it is fun work.

As a heart patient, there are going to be down times. My heart has palpitated all night, and I've woken up not feeling quite right. I need to decide in that moment if I'm going to call my doctor and cry or if I can do something to regain my sense of calm. Maybe my body is telling me I need rest today. I can tell when my body needs rest and I listen. I make sure that I am kind to myself.

Just start doing the simple things I have shared in this chapter, and soon you will get to a place where you feel more confident. You will get a sense of power, and you will know that you are no longer a victim of your condition. It's huge, and I know you can get there.

You are the average of 5 people you hang out with on a regular basis. I am really selective about who I associate with. Not in a snotty way. I pick the people that I let into my tribe. You operate under the vibe of your tribe which is why I never hung out with other heart patients at support groups.

I hung out with people that I wanted to model myself after. As a heart patient, make sure you are surrounded with people who lift you up. When you feel better, you can start taking steps like going to a class at the gym. You will find that your life will start changing and your wins will far outweigh the challenges you are facing.

It has been so long since I have perceived myself as a victim that most people don't even know I have such a serious heart condition. When I told some of my really close clients that I was writing this book they were amazed to find out what it was about because they never knew I had a heart condition. I no longer see myself as a heart patient, and that is what I want for you as well. I know you can get there and I am here to show you the way.

Chapter 6

Creating a New Relationship with Your Doctor and Professionals

EXPANDING YOUR PERCEPTION of yourself when you have a heart condition is absolutely essential if you want to live a normal life. No one is suggesting that you have to stop at normal because you can always shoot for exceptional if you want. But it is constant work to keep your focus on the things you want to be, do and have in your life and managing the limitations of your condition.

When you are living with a heart condition, you are constantly managing relationships. There is your relationship with yourself, what you want in life and what you believe is possible for you. Then there is your relationship to your condition and the limitations that it imposes on how you do things. There are the relationships with the people in your life and how they treat you because of the disease. Finally, there is the all-important relationship with your doctor and team of health professionals who tell you what you can and cannot do because of your condition.

After getting a handle on your mindset and your perception of yourself concerning what's going on with your heart, it is critical that you establish a healthy relationship with your specialist. This is not something that happens on its own, and if you leave it in their hands, you will likely stay stuck in fear of your condition and feeling like there is nothing you can do. This certainly is not their intention, but they are very busy and mostly concerned with making sure you don't die. But if you want to live a life full of all the things you want, then you must take charge of this relationship.

One thing that you can count on in life is change. Your condition is going to change, and you are going to have to shift your perception of yourself, what you can do and and how you go about living your life. This is not a bad thing, but again, if you don't take charge of your mindset and directing your focus, it is easy to fall back into the fear and doubt. Living with a heart condition, is not easy and you have to be on top of it, so you don't get paralyzed by the fear.

As I write this book, I am dealing with a change in my condition which means I have to manage all these relationships again. The night before I had to drive into Calgary to get threshold tests and muga scans done, I did not sleep well. I had butterflies the morning of. My mind was racing, and I just kept thinking, "now what are they going to do? Are they going to throw more drugs at me?" I have never been on meds, and I don't want to be, but we can't keep having these shocks happening. I am having ventricular tachycardias, which are life-threatening heart rhythms that we have to manage. The fear is back.

I thought I had gotten through the worst of everything

and could live a normal, healthy life, but I just got thrown another curve ball. At times like this I stay focused on my mindset because I know that if the fear takes over, it is almost impossible to overcome. I know there is always something I can do if I just stay open to the possibilities. I'll just duck so the curveball misses me or stand up and catch it.

I am blessed that my husband is so supportive and also into the power of the mind. The night before my tests, he found an article on the internet explaining about manifestation through the power of the heart energy. This article was very helpful in understanding the importance of focusing your mind and how your emotional state can affect heart health.

I was full of apprehension. The nurse had thrown out an idea about what could be going on with my heart and what they might do. The thoughts were just festering in my mind, and I needed to make sure that bad thoughts did not take root and grow. I didn't like the feeling of uncertainty because I felt like I had mastered the problem, but I know that it is just time for me to take the next step and I cannot do it in fear.

I'm not even really scared. It's more like WTF. I can understand how people can get beaten down, but it's learning to stand up again that's important. I am anticipating that they are going to take away things that I like to do again. I love getting up early and working out. It's not for everyone but for me it's a mental thing. It's my booster juice for the morning. Right now I can't do it, and I feel like I'm back in a fog again.

For me, I know that it is time to shift my paradigms again. There is always fear and apprehension when you do that, so I'm hoping for a new result. Not wishing. I am actively deciding how I want my result to look. I don't want to hear what I can't do anymore. I know what I want to be able to do and now we have to see how we are going to make this work. Which brings me back to managing the relationship with your doctor.

The hardest thing that cardiac specialists have to deal with among their patients are the fears and lack of motivation. For the most part, the patient is their own biggest limitation. Dr. Steven Sears brought this to light for me when we spoke about my experience with my condition at the event held in Calgary for people living with ICDs. I shared my story with Dr. Sears about how I live a normal life and do all the activities I do, and I was shocked by the response from other people living with devices and listening to all their limitations. I was awestruck by how people were so crippled by their conditions. Perhaps me living with this for the past 40 years, I had grown up with the limitations and my mindset was different towards my condition.

Rather than having a room full of people inspired by the hope and possibility that existed for every one of them with having this "safety net" of a device, I was in disbelief of the opposition. Anytime something positive was said about them having a safety net and to feel protected, people would say, "Yeah but I can't cause my condition is different." People got up and spoke about their limitations. They focused on things like not having the energy to get up and eat breakfast. There was so much focus on the negative, not on the fact that they had a safety net in place to protect their lives.

Dr. Sears event opened my eyes. I had never been to an

event like this before, and I was not aware of the mindset that pervades heart patients and people with ICDs. He told me that the biggest challenge I face is when I talk about what is possible. I need to start at a kindergarten level. Otherwise, these people won't be able to relate to me at all. In his studies, he developed a model for people who want to live a full life with a heart condition. It is simply that you must keep calm and take a step forward. People aren't calm. They lack focus on what is good and what is working. They have all this chatter about what they can't do, and they don't see the possibilities.

So let's talk about how to start living a full life despite your condition.

The first thing that you need to do is to get a determination of the seriousness of your condition.

What are the possibilities for any kind of activity within the limitations of your level of heart block and condition? I know exactly what my condition is. I have congenital heart block, and I am 100 percent dependent on my device.

Regular heart patients don't really ask what is going on. They just let their busy specialist get them in and out of their office as fast as possible. Don't let this happen. Without the understanding of your condition, you can't move forward. You need to know what you can do.

Make a list of your questions and bring it in with you to your appointment. People tend to forget everything they want to discuss when they are in the doctor's office. You have to be able to feel comfortable talking to your doctor. You have to get them talking to you in your language and speaking to you in a way that makes you understand. Get them to explain it in terms you understand and keep asking until you get it. It is your right to know exactly what is going on inside your body. Fear comes from lack of understanding.

When the doctors first told me I had dilated cardiomyopathy, I was clueless as to what that was. I asked him to help me understand what it meant. Dr. Exner got a plastic heart model and took it apart and showed me what was happening in my heart. He spent over an hour in the clinic with me explaining my condition. I feel it is of utmost importance to have a relationship with your Dr. in which you trust them with your life. I always feel empowered after an appointment with Dr. Exner. Most importantly, I have total faith and trust in him.

Not everyone is going to want to do what I do, but I know that they want something more than what they are living. Take the baby steps. Ask the doctor what your future looks like. What are things that you could do that would not cause you harm? Get the list of your possibilities.

Some people are given devices because they are in complete heart failure. Their condition may be a lot graver than mine, but there is still something they can do that gives them more quality of life.

Ask the doctor for the possibilities of what your life could look like. What can you absolutely not do? What are some things that you could do instead? What could your activity level look like? What would the doctor like it to look like? What could trigger an adverse reaction with your condition? Get to know your condition and your body so that you can work with it to expand your possibilities.

Dr. Exner told me that he was confident that I knew my body well enough. This happened because I asked the questions above and I experimented in the realm of what my doctors told me was safe. Every time I did something I felt better and found out that more was possible. It was so rewarding and freeing! I no longer felt trapped by my condition.

I didn't just go from having my pacemaker installed to snow skiing and water skiing. I took the baby steps. It's just that I have come so far that I can hardly remember not doing all the things I love to do. Dr. Exner just did not want me to put stress on the lead wire to my device. He was a bit scared of skiing because of what a fall could do, but he never said no don't do it.

Just take a small step and start to explore the area of possibility. It is the place where all the things that would make life more fun and fulfilling exist. I know it may seem like there is nothing you can do and that your condition is different, but I assure you that you will get hooked once you start taking baby steps.

Ask your questions. There aren't any stupid. Come on! We're talking about your heart. They need to answer you because it could mean life or death. You don't want to take that chance, and they don't either. I asked all my questions, and I am going in now to ask a whole bunch of new ones.

When I first got Dr. Exner as a specialist, I asked him why I was demand paced and now I am fully paced. Why did I have a pacemaker and now I have a defibrillator? He explained that when people have been full time paced for so many years and the way they placed the wires let the heart get weak on the left side ventricle. He explained his strategy of adding a third lead wire to the other side of the heart to strengthen it. It worked! I went from a low ejection fraction in the 30s to a mid-level ejection fraction in the 40s which would not even require and ICD.

I'm faced with uncertainty again because now my condition is becoming an arrhythmia issue. It's time for more questions and finding a theory about why this is happening and how we are going to handle it from here. To me, this is all just possibility, and I only expect life to get better from here!

Chapter 7

Creating Your New Personal Prognosis

WHEN I WAS first diagnosed with Congenital Heart Block, I was only 12 years old. So, the heart specialist and I never talked about my condition. Any explanation that he did give was directed to my parents, and they were just concerned with protecting me and keeping me safe. All I knew was that there was something very wrong with my heart, that I could not do what I wanted to do and that I could die at any moment.

What was my prognosis? I was told that I would be dependent on this device inside me for the rest of my life. I could not run or play sports, and whenever I exerted myself even a little bit, I would get dizzy and feel sick. I was not normal. I was fragile, and I hated being different. I didn't know about my life expectancy, I wasn't sure what activity was safe for me, and I was afraid to try anything.

Although I did not know it at the time, my entire focus was on making sure that my heart was beating and then trying to figure out whether I would have a bad day or not. I did not know about the power of my mind or the impact that my fear-based focus was having on my condition. All I knew was that I was not happy and I wanted to do more than I was doing.

Unfortunately, everyone around me was so intent on keeping me safe, that they would not let me try anything. While I know that they had the best of intentions at the time, I can now see that being this protected kept me from knowing my body and learning how to work with it. I was stuck in a cycle of negative, fear-based focus that left me feeling hopeless and depressed about my future. My fears were reinforced by developments in my condition. Almost dying when my device quit took away any confidence I had that it would keep me alive.

I know now when I look back at this time frame, that my thoughts and focus were attracting more problems and things to be fearful of into my reality. I also know that when I took control of my thoughts, my reality began to shift. While I can't pinpoint the exact moment when the shift in my mindset happened, I do know that as I began to care more and more about what I thought about, the more my condition and my life improved.

When I was old enough to move out on my own, things really changed for me. I was free to think for myself and make my own decisions, and this was very powerful. I was much less under the influence of my parents and the fears of other people so I could make choices that I would not have been allowed to make. I found myself thinking for the first time in my life that maybe I could do some of the things I dreamed of doing. Or at least I could try to find a way to do them.

When you are diagnosed with a heart condition and are

living with limitations, it can feel like you have no say in what you can or cannot do. It is very easy to become influenced by all the things that your doctor and the medical support staff tell you that you cannot do and become hopeless. I've done it myself, and I think it is so sad when people become complacent and give up on their dreams and desires. That's why it is so important to create a new prognosis for yourself. Your body may have limitations that are very real, but the limitations in your mind are not. You can change the thoughts you think. It just takes some practice, but I guarantee you it is worth it.

When I first became aware of the power of the mind, my whole life changed. I must have read the book, "The Power of Your Subconscious Mind" by Joseph Murphy 10 times! I was amazed that there was something I could do to change my life despite the limitations imposed on me by my condition. I highly recommend getting a copy of this book.

The most amazing thing was when I started concentrating and doing work with the power of my mind, I began to see how much more potential I had in my body. I had been living in so much fear and doubt because I had always lived in the unknown and I did not see any possibilities for the future. Working with my mind gave me something that I could count on even when my body was limiting me. It made me want to find something better that worked for me. What amazed me most was how much better I felt!

So where do you start? The first thing you need to do to begin tapping into the power of your mind is to calm your thoughts. Just as Dr. Sears told me that most heart patients lack calmness of mind, this is the biggest thing that gets in the way of them being able to use this amazing power to feel better. I know that it can seem like being calm is almost impossible to do when you're worried about your heart and whether it will support you or not but you just have to try it and see. I promise that you will be amazed.

How do you stop all that monkey chatter that's going on in there? You know, that commentary about everything you see and do. All the opinions and beliefs that just keep running in there on autoplay. It can drive you crazy! Just spend a little time listening to it to see how ridiculous it actually is. You might find yourself getting annoyed or even angry. It's good to know that you have this perpetual background noise going on in your head and how emotionally riled up it can get you. That in itself should give you some incentive to want to calm it down.

The beginner meditation that I shared in the last chapter is the perfect tool to use to introduce that sense of stillness to your mind and body. It instructs you in how to sit and guides you to focus your attention and breath. While this meditation worked really well for me, everyone has their own personal preference. Try it out and see how you like it. I must have tried at least ten different ones before I found this one. You just need to find one where the person's voice and the music resonate with you. If you search beginner meditation on youtube, you will find tons of videos. You can even get as specific as "Meditative practices when suffering from heart conditions." You'll be amazed by what comes up.

You Get What You Focus On

I'm big into the Law of Attraction. I must have watched

the movie, "The Secret" 30 times. I totally believe that what you think about, you bring about. Your thoughts create your reality. That's why the first step in creating your new prognosis is all about calming your mind. You need to get a handle on what thoughts you are thinking. Just even knowing that you are having thoughts is a big step. At least once you realize that you don't like the thoughts that you are having, you can decide that you want to do something about them.

The biggest problem with being diagnosed with a heart condition is everything that you are told is negative. You are told about what doesn't work in your body and what you can no longer do. You are warned about all the activities that are now dangerous to you. They tell you what foods to avoid because they are bad for you. With all this focus on things that are negative, it is next to impossible to appreciate anything good.

We may have ourselves convinced that there is nothing good about this situation to appreciate but I want to tell you how wrong that assumption is. Just the simple fact that you are alive right now means that infinitely more is going right inside you than is going wrong. The problem is that we just don't take any time to acknowledge the things that are working and be grateful for them. Think about it. Are you breathing? Do you have to tell your lungs to work? Thank God you don't, or you would have all your mental capacity taken up with making sure that you didn't stop. And what would you do when you fell asleep?

A belief is just a thought that you keep thinking and rethinking. Our focus on it becomes so strong that we actually bring it into existence. Our thoughts have the power to manifest when we hold them in steady focus so what we believe tends to come true for us. The big problem is that when we are afraid of something, we focus on it a lot. Worrying about something that you fear is pretty much like praying for it to happen.

I really want to emphasize how important it is for you to clean up your thoughts and make sure that they are positive. Most of us go around with our heads packed with negative thoughts and then we complain about how nothing ever goes our way. We are always talking about how things went from bad to worse. If anything I am saying makes any sense to you, you should be seeing that thinking this way not only makes your mood worse, but it makes your body feel terrible. Fortunately, the opposite is also true.

Get the movie, "The Secret". Watch it more than once. I find that every time I watch it, I pull something new from it. As you're watching it, see if you can relate any of it to your life circumstances. There is always some aspect of your life that will resonate. It will start to give you a sense of how you see yourself. That's why movies and literature can be so helpful. They can give you the tools and exercises that will reveal your self-image. Often you find a scientific explanation of what is going on inside you.

Dr. Murphy's book is very powerful, and a must read. More about why this book had such an impact on you………..

If you have read this far, I am going on the assumption that you are willing to do something to improve your life despite your condition. You are wanting to start living again and reawaken your desires. I am sharing my story to show you what worked for me. I know that if you apply what you find in this book, it will work for you too. It will also lead you on the path towards more things that will help you live a great life regardless of what is going on with your heart. When you start seeking solutions, more and more options start to present themselves. Like attracts like. This is why it is so important to get out of a negative headspace.

You have to understand that your thoughts are your point of attraction. If you are only seeing the problems in everything and not noticing what is going right, you are only going to attract more of what is not working. This cascades into your emotions and your body. Unhealthy thoughts lead to an unhealthy mind and body.

Try this exercise for 30 days. Get up every morning and write down a list of things that you appreciate about other people, yourself, your life and even your doctor. Aim for ten things you appreciate every day. In 30 days the difference in your emotional state will astound you. I can guarantee you that you will feel a difference in your body too. But I can't just explain this to you. You have to actually do it to know what I mean. Another powerful tool is to stand in front of your mirror every morning and smile. Just simply. Stand there and smile at your reflection. I am a happy person. Smiling and making people laugh makes me feel so good, it's the best mood booster ever. Laughter is and always will be the best therapy for any disease. I have found in the past 40 years of dealing with my cardiac condition that making other people laugh and smile makes my emotional state and well being so much better.

I still get moments where I am sucked into the negative, but I feel my lows much less intensely now. I know what

my triggers are and I can pull myself out of them quickly.
At times when my condition is uncertain, and I can't do
my regular workouts, it is easy for me to dip down into the
"here I go again" attitude. If I don't catch it, I can downward spiral into hopelessness and depression, so it is a must
for me to pull myself out quickly. Anyone can get caught
up in that sort of downward momentum. Learning your
triggers and developing strategies to pull yourself back up
is life changing.

Our best friend was diagnosed with glioblastoma, a
cancerous brain tumor and he was given a year to live. My
husband and I got him doing the power of the mind work
because we regularly hung out with him and his wife. Typ-
ically patients with this diagnosis have a 15 month survival
time. With his strength and positive determination, he sur-
passed that time frame by a few years. What else is possible?
When you're terminal, what have you got to lose? Celebrate
every small victory and surprise yourself! Make a committed decision and demand it of yourself. It WORKS every
time!

I have another friend who was diagnosed with cancer
shortly after the birth of her son. She was not supposed to
live to see his first birthday but she just celebrated his 18th!
She's having more issues right now, but if she chooses her
focus and keeps her mind full of positive thoughts, who
knows how many more of his birthdays she'll see?

The mind is like a garden with very rich soil. Anything
can grow abundantly well in it, and that's just the problem.
If you don't tend to it, the weeds get a hold and overgrow it.
If you want to grow a beautiful garden it takes planting the

right seed, love and care and a lot of weeding. You want to pull the bad thoughts out of your mind just like you pluck weeds from your garden. You need to plant good thoughts and water them with appreciation and attention, so they grow up big and strong. Then the good thoughts take hold of the garden and make it hard for the weeds to take root.

I have been interested in personal growth and the power of the mind for over 25 years now, and it's a lot like bathing. You need to make it a regular habit. You can't just do it when you feel like it or when you think you need it. If you don't bathe daily, well, you get the point. If you don't do your personal development every day, your mind starts to stink. Consistency is vital to success.

No matter what the situation is inside you or around you, you can always focus on the positive.

Most people only seem to focus on and talk about the negative. We have been trained this way by the media, the news, and magazines. The negative gets more of a reaction from us. It gets us emotionally riled up, and it sells magazines. Just check out the magazine rack at the grocery store, and you'll see who is cheating, dying, suing someone for millions or stabbing someone in the back. It's up to you to block that out and learn to appreciate the good in everything.

My spa is in a very nice area of town. Just across the way is an establishment that has always been a bar or nightclub. The owner has always been a good businessman, and the patrons of his business have never caused any disturbance to my shop because we operate at completely different hours. The local news station showed up at my spa wanting to interview me about my opinion about the fact that it was becoming a strip club. Now I don't support that type of establishment, but I don't choose to focus my energy against anything either. When they interviewed me I just said that as long as he was following all regulations, I did not care but if all the businesses in town chose to uplift each other, think about how successful we'd all be. In their story, they only quoted me as saying that he had better follow all the regulations. The negative is what sells.

People react to the negative because it is sensational and gets a reaction. You have to be careful what you let in. It's up to you to start finding the positive in everything that you observe. It is so easy to get sucked into a negative downward spiral. That's why most people live like that, and it causes sickness. You can change your vibration by starting to find the positive even if it's really small.

Decide now that you want to get the positive mindset. Start focusing on what you do want to see around you and in your life. My whole life changed when I started to change the way that I viewed myself. I changed my mind about how I wanted to live, and I decided to want to change my results. To my amazement, I started to feel better physically, and my body began to change.

You have to decide how you want to feel and know that what you are currently living is not how you are going to live.

Stop focusing on what you have and start focusing on what you want to see in your life. Simple exercises like writing positive things down in a journal can be such an easy way to get a positive vibration in your life. It is amazing how good it makes you feel. You will find yourself starting to smile more, and you can't stay angry if you start smiling. Look in the mirror and start smiling at yourself every day. Smile at more people. It changes your mood.

When I walk into my spa and have another 12 hour day, I can't say that I wouldn't rather be the one in the chair getting a spa service. I make a shift and start smiling and joking, and it is all good. My energy stays high all day, and my customers see my happy positive attitude. They ask if I ever have a bad day. I don't because I decided a long time ago that a day was not worth wasting. It changes my mood, my health, and my life.

You get a domino effect, and it ripples into other parts of your life. You start to forget about the other stuff that you don't want to focus on. Once you start seeing a positive result, it creates the excitement to want to try more. If you go to the gym and stick with it, you start seeing results.

You start telling people and wanting to do more.

Committing yourself to something positive and happy every day, no matter how small, will keep you focused and motivated in a positive way. You will start thinking of more good things to do, and you will attract more good things. Good things will start to come to you out of the blue.

You will start seeing the next step that you did not even think was possible. You will start taking new actions that you never dreamed you would take. New people will show up in your life and show you new things that you never thought of before. The path towards your desires will start to show up in front of you.

As you start moving towards the goal, the goal starts moving towards you. Once you decide to move towards something better, new little avenues open up and make it possible to get to where you want to go. Surround yourself with like-minded people who support you in what you want to see in your life. Bob Proctor, one of my mentors, teaches that you should surround yourself with the six people that you most admire. Identify the characteristics that you most like in them and model yourself after them.

Don't focus on your limitations. It's important to talk to your doctor and find out what you can do. You may have to modify how you go about an activity, but you will find a way to make it work.

Right now I can't train the way that I am used to until my doctors figure out how to get my heart rhythm back under control. I have been shocked twice by my defibrillator, and they don't know why. I asked my specialist Dr. Exner for a list of things that I can and cannot do so that my trainer feels comfortable working with me. All I know is that I am no longer allowed to do interval training or to squat 100 pound weights.

Dr. Exner got in touch with my trainer, and his first comment was that he was not used to writing this kind of a letter. Most people ask him to write them letters excusing them from activities and duties.

In the next chapter, we will walk step by step through my system for creating the life that you want. It's all a mind game. It takes work, but the work is all an inside job. When you start to believe that things can change for you, they start to change. It all starts with belief.

Wayne Dyer

"Most people think you will believe it when you see it but, you need to believe it before you see it."

Chapter 8

Designing the Action Plan that is Right for You

THIS CHAPTER IS about creating an action plan to create what you want on your terms. It's about getting from where you are now with your heart condition to living, doing and being the person you want to be in the life you want to live. The stories that I have shared about my life are about me doing what I had to do to build a life I love. You may like some of the things I have created and you may not. It's your life, and you get to choose.

I'm not going to tell you all the information you've heard over and over from the heart institute about what you should and shouldn't do. We already know that we need to eat healthily and exercise. Tell me something I don't know. Don't worry. I'm not going to make you start doing all the things that you don't want to do. In this chapter, my goal is to get you to want to do things that make you feel better. I want you to get excited about your life and want to see something different.

I have to admit that because I was diagnosed when I was 12, things were a lot different for me than for someone who is diagnosed in adulthood. My understanding of my condition and of life, in general, was through the eyes of a little girl who just wanted to play and be normal. I didn't understand what the doctor was saying, and I didn't like being fragile and afraid that I was going to die. All I know is that being different meant that I got bullied in school and I was hell-bent on not being different.

I have been doing my own thing and telling my doctor how it is for so long that I can't imagine not doing things that way. It took some deep introspection to come up with the steps that I took to create the action plan that I have for living my life on my terms. Many of the things that I did to gain freedom in my life despite my condition just seemed like a logical step for me at the time, and I didn't think anything of them. Most of the work is inner work and has to do with overcoming fear. I still study this every day, and it has been so rewarding in every aspect of my life. I know it will be for you as well.

If you have read this far, I am assuming that you are ready to do what it takes to reclaim your power in your life. We all have to get to this point before we can make any changes in our lives that stick. I'm going to help you design your own personal action plan so that you can take baby steps towards your goal. I want it to be so simple that everything in your action plan just seems like the next logical step for you.

Below are the steps to creating your life on your terms despite your heart condition. These are the steps that I used to change my own life, and now I walk people with heart conditions through them so they can break out of the fear and doubt and start taking action towards the life they want to live.

1. Start where you are

2. Decide what you want in your life without worrying about how you will get it

3. Take any action no matter how small to make yourself feel better

4. Celebrate every small victory

5. Ask yourself what the next logical step may be and then take it

You might be thinking that this looks too simplistic to be effective but bear with me. I used these steps to go from being a fragile little 12-year-old who would get dizzy if she walked too fast to being able to squat 125 pounds in the gym and do wind sprints and burpees. I can also work on my feet 12 hours a day and still walk my dogs and take care of my acreage. When I was 12, I was just wondering how long I would live. Now I just keep looking for new and exciting things that I want to do in my life.

Everyone has their own wants and desires. What I have in my life is what I wanted and desired when I felt like I was incapable of having it. By making these five steps a regular practice, I created the life I wanted and continue to do so. You can do this too. On your own terms. I'll walk you through the steps.

Step 1-Start Where You Are

There really is no other place that you need to be. It does not matter what you could do or what you were like before your diagnosis. The key is acceptance of what is. What is right now? There is nothing wrong with where you are unless you decide that you have a problem with it. When you can get to the place of acceptance that where you are in the now is okay without feeling mad about how things used to be or stressed out by how you think things should be, you have reached acceptance. This is the only starting point that is possible for creating the life that you want.

Acceptance cannot be confused with complacency or giving up. You are not saying that you are broken and that this is as good as it's going to get. You are simply acknowledging that this is where you are right now and that it is what it is. Once you see things as they really are, you can make decisions from a place of nonresistance. It does not mean that you want to stay where you are. It simply means that you can see and appreciate that where you are is the starting point and that you can feel good knowing that from there, you can get to anywhere you want to go.

For me, the acceptance came when I realized that no matter how much I wanted to be normal, I still had a device that kept my heart beating. If I overexerted myself, I would get dizzy and feel sick. That was what I was dealing with. If I wanted to "not be different," I was going to have to find some way to do it within these parameters. Wishing that my life was the way it was before I was diagnosed only made me feel worse. Hiding at my grandma's and feeling sorry for myself just made me depressed. It wasn't until I started to appreciate how much my friends wanted to include me and how hard some teachers worked to help me participate that I started to find more ways to be normal.

My first form of gratitude came when I would say my

prayers at night. When I would ask God to bless the people in my life, I would start to think about the things that I appreciated about them. I would drift off to sleep thinking about how caring and supportive my parents, friends, and teachers were and how much better my life was because of that. I felt so much better doing that than when I would focus on the things that I could no longer do and how much I missed being able to play sports. I would wake up with more energy and have a better day whenever I practiced gratitude at night.

I never miss my gratitude practice. In fact, every night I write down ten new things I am grateful for. This is a must for creating acceptance in your life. It is so much easier to start where you are when you are grateful. This practice of gratitude keeps you focused on always finding more things to appreciate and it opens you up to all the possibilities that exist despite your diagnosis or condition.

Ten Things that I Am Grateful for Today:

1.

2.

3.

4.

5.

6.

7.

8.

9.

10.

Step 2-Decide What You Want In Your Life Without Worrying About How You Will Get It

It can be very difficult to set goals that seem unattainable when you can't see a way of reaching them. Especially when you have been diagnosed with a heart condition. It seems like you're always being told what you can't do and all the things that are no longer an option for you. I know how it is. You can find yourself feeling like your life is over and that there is no point in wanting or hoping for anything because it is never going to happen.

Unfortunately, this type of thinking is exactly what keeps people stuck where they are and miserable. It creates an ever-expanding fear barrier that becomes impossible to see beyond or break through. That's why we need to keep Step 2 light and easy. You can't let worrying about how you're going to make your goal happen to stop you from wanting it to happen. We just want to get more desire and eagerness in our lives for things that we don't have yet. We don't need to know how it's going to come about but we do need to get our mind looking for possibilities.

The law of attraction always works. Whatever you are focusing on comes to you more and more. If you keep focusing on what you can no longer do or have, you will find that more and more things you want will become unavailable to you. And that's no fun at all. But if you focus on the excitement and the feeling you will have when you are doing or enjoying something that you really want in your life, the law of attraction will bring you ways to get it. Your mind will start to focus on the opportunities that are all around you but that you just have not been paying attention to and that will lead you to the next step.

What are five things that you would do if you had no fear or limitations in your life?

1.

2.

3.

4.

5.

Step 3-Take Any Action No Matter How Small To Make Yourself Feel Better

When you begin to understand that the law of attraction always works, you get more picky about the thoughts you choose to think. Steps 1 and 2 naturally start to direct your thoughts in a positive direction which gets the law of attraction working to bring you more of what you do want in your life rather than making day to day events and your condition slide downhill.

Adding more appreciation and acceptance to your life and allowing yourself to want new things in your experience starts to direct your mind towards all the possibilities and opportunities that you may not have been seeing. You may find yourself having thoughts about trying something that you may think is absurd. Just sit with the thought and let your mind play with it. If you are thinking of trying something that just seems out of the question, ask yourself how you could make it work. Is there something similar or scaled down that you could do instead?

When I wanted to start working out, I asked my friend who was an aerobics instructor if I could just hang out at the back of her class and do whatever I could do. I gave myself permission to sit out of exercises that I found too hard and if it got to be too much. I was at the back of the class. I wouldn't disturb anyone if I snuck out. I amazed myself by getting through the whole class. It wasn't a star performance, but at least I did something.

It isn't a matter of accomplishing anything big. You simply want to take an action that is different from what you usually do on a daily basis. Your actions start to generate new outcomes in your life and change the course of the possibilities that present themselves to you. The actions start to create energy and make you feel like you can do something. Because the truth of the matter is that there is always some small action that you can take. It may seem insignificant on its own, but we are not concerned about the individual action itself. It is the power of the sum of a week of tiny, easy, almost effortless actions that turn into results. When you keep this up, you start to notice momentum building. It generates more energy, enthusiasm and desire. Law of attraction starts showing you even more opportunities to get what you want and all you have to do is take the next step.

Every morning, review your gratitude list and your list of five things that you would like in your life. Ask yourself what small actions you could take today that would move you closer to having or experiencing what you want in your life. Write your action ideas down so you can see them.

Three Possible actions that I could take today to get me closer to my goal are:

1.

2.

3.

Another possibility could be:

Ask if you could do one of those actions today. If it does not seem possible, ask yourself what you could do instead and add the action that you come up with to the list as another possibility.

For example, you may have decided that you want to start eating a healthier diet. Maybe you thought an action could be to eat healthy today or make a healthy meal. I want you to choose an action that is so easy for you to achieve that you can't not do it. Making a meal may be hard. Maybe you don't have the right food in your house. Perhaps you don't even know what you need. An action that would be really easy to take could be just to research some easy ways to make your diet healthier. That could be your one action today. Following up on one of the ways to make your diet healthier could be your action tomorrow or the next day.

Commit to taking one action from the list today and do it. In the evening, when you are doing your gratitude practice, add the action you took to your gratitude list because being able to take action is always something to be grateful for! If you didn't get it done, ask yourself how you could make it easier to do tomorrow, and you'll be amazed by how many new possibilities will come up.

Step 4-Celebrate Every Small Victory

Once you get into a rhythm of taking small daily actions, you will quickly notice the momentum and energy that begins to build in your life. You will feel an excitement and enthusiasm beginning to infuse your outlook. Most of all, you will start to see things happening and changing in your life.

At first, it may not seem like much. You may think that you are so far away from getting what you want or achieving your goal. The key is to keep your focus in the right place. Where you are is on the way to getting what you want. That is why it is so important to be where you are in Step 1. But if you have been focusing on what you want and taking small daily actions, it is impossible to be in the same place you were yesterday or last week.

You want to make a big deal about the changes that you start to see in your life. If for example, in your decision to eat healthier, you discovered that you could substitute Greek yogurt for some heavier, creamier foods and you have started to enjoy doing it, celebrate! You are eating healthier than you were last week. What else is possible now? Add your celebration to your gratitude practice every night.

Step 5-Ask Yourself What the Next Logical Step May Be and Then Take It

As you start to celebrate your daily victories, you will notice that they begin to add up fast. The goals that you set and the things that you once thought were impossible may look a lot closer on the horizon than they once appeared. You might find yourself feeling like you now think that they are more achievable and that you even know the path to take.

It doesn't matter if you still don't know how to get there. You just need to keep applying these five steps. Step 5 is simply to ask yourself what the next logical step could be. This just keeps you moving towards your goal and attracting more possibilities to help you get there.

You will find that people will show up on your path and they will show you shortcuts that you would never have found if you did not start taking action. You will be at the right place at the right time to see or hear something that gives you the perfect idea for a solution to a problem you had. You will get emails and advertisements that offer exactly what you were searching for. It will just seem like everything is lining up to help you get to your goal.

For me, after I found that I could get through an aerobics class, I wanted to do more. Soon I found myself wanting to take a course to be an instructor. I just thought it would be cool to be a fitness instructor with a pacemaker. I never thought about what it would mean to teach.

The momentum starts to become unstoppable. You may reach your goal, or you may find that you get somewhere different that is even better. You couldn't have known this without taking action. For me, I found that I loved physical fitness. I had many limitations to work around, but I would not have met the people who are in my life now or get the amazing support that I have gotten if I did not decide to try my friend's class. The doctors who have worked with me to get the right devices that can support my activity would not have shown up. Now I have Dr. Exner who fights for me and has performed specialized procedures just because he knows that I insist on being able to perform at a high physical level.

You may not want this in your life, but I guarantee you that you can have what you want in your life. You just need to use the power of your mind and get the law of attraction working to create what you want. Spend time with these five steps. Make them a daily practice in your life and I promise you that you will be emailing me the most amazing results!

Chapter 9

Creating Your New Self Image

THE WAY YOU see yourself in life is powerful. It can help you to live a life of joy and freedom or one of misery and confinement. Self-image has been so impactful in my life and has made it possible for me to live a "normal life," despite the serious obstacles posed by my condition. I have been through the ups and downs of a good self-image and a bad self-image and have experienced the immediacy of the results in how much I enjoyed any given day.

I know that it can be hard to think that life is grand and that you have every opportunity in the world when you are diagnosed with something as serious as a heart condition. Any life-threatening diagnosis is a serious issue, and we immediately become hyper-vigilant to what's happening in our bodies. We are no longer the person we used to be before the diagnosis when we were "healthy," and we take on a new "sick" persona.

We start to identify with our condition, and it begins to shape everything we do. Because your whole life is being seen through the lens of your condition, you observe the events and circumstances differently. You start projecting your condition onto what is going on around you. The limitations of your conditions become limitations on your life, and it is hard not to feel like you are damaged, different and "less than."

My diagnosis came right before I entered my teenage years. It's bad enough trying to figure out who the heck you are when you are normal and healthy. I went from being normal one day to being sick and coming back to school a couple of months later as the fragile girl with the battery pack. Kids are merciless and the years between 13 and 18 were the most horrific years of my life.

The self-image that resulted was very low. While the other girls' bodies were developing and they were wearing stylish clothes, I was physically scarred with a battery the size of a cigarette pack on my stomach. I had to wear unfashionable, frumpy outfits and I would never look good in a bikini. People either made fun of me or felt sorry for me. School was a place of bullying, and I just wanted to escape. My safe place was my grandma's house, and I would go there at lunch to get a reprieve and feel loved.

At home, I looked happy, but I never shared my feelings. My parents were doing everything they could to make sure I had a good life. My condition had caused a lot of stress in the family and put them through a big financial strain. I felt responsible, and this made me beat myself up. I didn't want to trouble them with what was happening at school. It would just get brushed off anyway.

My dad grew up in Holland. The way we express our feelings today would never fly with him back then. He's a lot different now! Back then it was understood that we were to keep our feelings to ourselves and that we should know our parents are proud of us and love us. Today I make sure I share my love for my kids with them whenever I can, and I am always telling them how proud I am of them. One of my greatest accomplishments to date will now and always be how so very proud I am of my two amazing adult children, Justin and Sienna. They continue to inspire me. They are the best decision I have ever made. Life could not have always been easy for them, especially through the many peaks and valleys of my health issues, I am a survivor for them.... because of them.

Getting through my teenage years was all about survival both physically and emotionally. I'd wake up every morning and take my pulse to see if my heart was okay. I wanted to know if I was going to have a good day or a bad day. I also just wanted to feel good about myself, so I would make myself find something good to focus on in my life. A lot of the time I would picture my grandmother and my core group of friends that I knew cared about me and just let me be me.

I wanted so badly to be "normal," but my condition just made it impossible. I would be so mad at my life, and I even found myself mad at God. Growing up my parents made us go to church every Sunday and Catechism class once a week after school. I just could not reconcile how a God that loved me so much could let me live like this. But wanting to find a reason or someone to blame did not make me feel one bit better about myself. I would only get more miserable and feel even more powerless.

So I accepted that I needed to do what I needed to do to

feel good. And that was to focus on people and things that made me feel happy and not think about the other stuff that made me feel bad. I learned that my condition was just a set of circumstances that I had to contend with but that feeling happy was something I had control over. When I felt angry, lonely and afraid, I just needed to think about having fun with a really good friend, and I would feel better. I found that doing this made it a lot easier to survive those years and could even generate some anticipation of better times to come.

Although I did not know it at the time, I was learning that self-image was a choice and a creation of your thoughts and decisions. I was just trying to keep happy, so I could get through another day of school, but my survival mechanism of pushing bad thoughts out of my head was training me to be a very positive person. I attracted some very loving people around me who appreciated this in me, and no matter what was going on around me, I could find a reason to be happy.

Building this positive focus muscle during my highschool years set me up for a huge life transformation when I graduated. Getting married and moving out of the house gave me a lot more freedom to make my own decisions and I really started to experience the creative and attractive power of positive thinking. More of what I wanted started to appear in my life. And then in my early 20s, I got my first dual chamber pacemaker, and my whole life opened up before my eyes! It felt like getting the new device was magic, but I know that if I did not have all those years of practice focusing my thoughts that it could easily have been something else to complain about.

Today, most people don't even know that I have a heart

condition or a device. People ask me if I ever have a bad day. I always feel good, I consider myself a happy person because I decided that was how I was going to live. My self-image has come a long way, and I love who I am.

Perception Is Everything

Two people can be in exactly the same situation and have completely opposite experiences. I can only imagine what someone getting their first device in their 30s, 40s or 50s would think and feel after perhaps a lifetime with a "normal" heart. When I got my first dual chamber pacemaker, it was life-changing. I had been paced at 72 bpm for so many years that if my heart rate varied just the slightest fraction of a beat, I would feel it and wonder what was happening. When I stood up after the surgery, and my heart started to speed up, I freaked out. The doctors had to calm me down and explain to me that this is how normal hearts work and my heart was going to work like normal now. No more getting dizzy with the slightest bit of exertion. I could participate in physical activity again! I felt like I got my life back. Someone else getting their first device could easily think that their life as they knew it had been taken away.

Whether the device is giving you your life back or taking it away is a matter of perception. For me, I kept wondering what else was possible and discovering how wonderful life could be. I would try new things and be surprised and delighted by the mere fact that I could actually do it. There were still things that I could not do because of the limitations of my condition, but I was so taken by what I could do that it did not matter. Somehow, I always seemed to push myself beyond my limitations and always found ways to do more than a typical heart patient would even consider trying.

I have noticed that a lot of people tend to focus on what they can't do and what is not working. This has a very negative impact on their perception of a situation. This also presents an opportunity to find something positive in the situation to focus on. Knowing that you can influence your perception by choosing where to focus and what to think about is powerful. Actually influencing your perception intentionally will alter the course of your life.

Use Your Power to Choose

Sometimes we can feel like life leaves us at a point where we have no choice. This is very common among people with heart conditions because of the dangers and limitations involved in the situation. However, having no choice is a self-imposed sentence that makes us feel like a victim. There is always a choice to make, and you always have the power to choose.

While you may not be able to physically participate in an activity because your body will not permit you to, you can choose what that means. If you decide that it means your life sucks and just mope, you have chosen to be a victim of the circumstance. However, you could choose to seek an opportunity to try something different or find a modification that would allow you to participate in some way.

Deciding that you have no choice and doing nothing is making a choice. The result is disempowering, and you end up feeling bad. Seeking opportunity leads to discovering something new. It also leads to options which give you even more choice. Finding a way to do something that you initially thought you could not do is empowering and makes you feel good.

I got really good at doing this as I found out that I was capable of more and more activities. It has gotten to the point where I am now constantly negotiating with my doctor about what I can do. I continually present him with new possibilities for doing activities until we find one that works.

Your Self-Image Is All Mindset

Your thoughts create your reality, and your body responds to your thoughts. Letting your thoughts do their own thing is dangerous and always leads to feeling bad. That's why it is so important to pay attention to what you are thinking and to make sure you are choosing your thoughts.

I only started to study mindset when I turned 50. I got really into it because I realized that I had been practicing it my whole life. The books I read only supported what I already knew. I had always been careful about what I allowed in my mind because I knew that thinking about the wrong things made my day really difficult. The average person can get away with bad thinking and only suffer from feeling bad emotionally. If I didn't watch my thoughts, I would suffer physically and feel sick on top of being in a bad mood. This was a blessing and a curse, but it did make me keep my mindset as clean as possible.

As a result, I was constantly looking for the good in situations, other people and myself. The more I appreciated the good around me and within me, the better and happier I felt. This helped me to see how powerful my mind was and want to use it more. I became curious, eager and confident about what I was capable of and this had huge impacts on my self-esteem.

No matter what is going on in your body and how out of control things around you may feel, you can always take charge of your mindset. Being a victim is detrimental to your self-image. Mastering your mindset is the way to make peace with your condition and create a self-image that makes you happy.

How to Create a Good Self Image Despite Your Condition

"There's a point in life where you need to stop reading other people's books and write your own."

Albert Einstein

My study of personal development and mindset has helped me to understand how I have come to terms with my heart condition and living with my device. I know that I could easily have spent my whole life being the fragile little girl my parents brought home from the hospital in 1977. My desire to be normal has become a reality, and now I am proud to be who I am. I can actually do things that normal people can't do.

Here are the simple steps to creating your new self image:

1. See Your Condition as It Is
2. Know that You Are Not Your Condition

3. Use The Power of Your Thoughts to Create Your Reality

4. Maintain Focus on What You Want and Acknowledge Every Small Win

5. Make Peace with Where You Are and Keep Creating with Focus

Step 1-See Your Condition As It Is

"It is what it is." This is such a great statement, but I don't think many people really mean it when they say it. Perception always influences how things appear, so it is much more accurate to say that, "It is what I perceive it to be."

The key to applying this statement to your condition successfully is to strip away any meaning that you have attached to experiencing it. There are so many levels of meaning to having a health condition. You may think that you are sick and disabled. You could see the condition as a limitation that makes you dependent on others. It may be the cause of the role you play in the relationships you have with others. The number of meanings that a heart condition could have is infinite, and there are even some positive ones.

In this step, we just want to try to see our heart condition for what it is. For me, my heart functions with the help of a device that regulates its rhythm and protects it from dangerous arrhythmias. If I am conscious of making sure that this device can function properly and respect the physical nature of its wires and connections, my heart basically functions like a normal heart.

Step 2-Know that You Are Not Your Condition

Most people identify themselves with a role they play at work, in a relationship or in society. You may see yourself as your occupation, as a parent, a taxpayer, an ethnicity or a citizen of a country, just to name a few. People with heart conditions see themselves as heart patients, and it does not help that the medical community refers to us as our conditions rather than the people we are. The truth is that you are a brilliant person who is here to create an amazing life. Anytime you accept the role of anything else; you distract yourself from who you really are and diminish how well you are attracting what you want in your life.

It is very important to see yourself as separate from your condition. This takes away the power that the condition has over you and gives you back your power as the creator of your own reality.

I used to get so mad when my parents would run into people they knew and introduce me as their daughter with the pacemaker. I'd be thinking to myself, "I have a name. It's Linda." And I would wonder who I would be if I didn't have a heart condition. All I could think was that I'd still be Linda, but I would do more things that I wanted to do. And that is exactly what happened.

Step 3-Use The Power Of Your Thoughts To Create Your Reality

The law of attraction states that what you think about, you bring about. We have something like 60,000 thoughts a day, but most of the time we are thinking the same thought.

That thought is sustaining the reality that you live in every day. If you love your life, then go ahead and keep thinking what you're thinking but if you don't, you're going to want to change what you are thinking.

Everything you think and say is a prayer, be it positive or negative. When you say a prayer, it's like you are talking to God. When you use your intuition, it's God talking to you. Pay attention to your thoughts and notice if you like what you are thinking. Are you thinking about the things you want in your life or do you keep focusing on the circumstances that you are living that you don't like? Focusing on the things that we don't like keeps them in our lives.

If you want something new in your life, you need to focus on what it would be like to already have it. To already be experiencing it. If thinking about what you want makes you feel bad because you don't have it, you're focusing on what you don't want, and that is what you will continue to attract.

I was so focused on wanting to be normal that I just did not accept that I wasn't. I was constantly looking for ways to do the things I wanted to do and thinking about how I could get my doctors and my parents to let me play the way other kids did. I always did find a way even if it did not look like what I had first expected. Now, for all intents and purposes, I am normal.

If you have trouble feeling happy or excited when you think about things that you want to have or do in your life, spending time in meditation will help. Meditation calms your mind and releases the hold that negative thoughts have over you. You will find that during and after a meditation, you will be more intuitive. It will be like God is telling you how to get what you want.

Step 4-Maintain Focus On What You Want And Acknowledge Every Small Win

Often, we are focused on things in our lives that are not going well and the stuff we want to change. For a long time, I could only see how horribly different my pacemaker made me from all the other kids. I would think about the teasing and bullying, and I would cry. I so wanted to be normal, but all I thought about was why I could not be. This made it impossible for the law of attraction to make my life normal.

Gradually, I started to be happy about the things in my life that did work. I liked going to my grandma's at lunch, and I felt better when I was there. I could avoid the kids that teased and bullied me and focus on being with my closest friends. Even if I could not always get away from the kids I did not like, I did not think about them when I got home. I would only think about my core group of friends and how lucky I was to have them.

Things did get better, and I would do my gratitude practice at night when I said my prayers. Little wins add up. Life got more and more normal. Now I am grateful for the struggles I had in school because I know I would not be living such a great life without them.

Step 5-Make Peace With Where You Are And Keep Creating Aith Focus

The biggest lesson that I learned from my heart condition and creating a great life despite it is that everything was always alright. Wherever I was, however hard I was struggling, I was always okay. I did not feel that way in the moment but looking back; I can see that I was.

I know this today and when I feel like I have a problem I tell myself that everything is alright. Even when I am frustrated or feel hopeless, I catch myself and make peace with where I am. Suddenly I regain my capacity to think about what I want, and I can see opportunities to get it.

Even today I get rattled by my condition from time to time. The defibrillator in my device has shocked me on two occasions while I was working out and I had to take some time off work and lost my Driver's license for a month while they try to figure out what's happening. I find my thoughts starting to go down the rabbit hole, and I stop them immediately. I am on beta blockers, and they make me feel awful. I want off them. They think that the shock may have created a neural pathway in my heart that is making it easier for these arrhythmias to happen. Now they want to do an ablation which is a surgery to disrupt that pathway, so this does not happen.

As for me, I am convinced that I will be off the medication and that I will create a new neural pathway in my heart, so I don't need the surgery. I'm back at the gym, and I feel good. That's a win for me. I know that I am okay and that everything always works out.

This is the continual cycle. You run into problems. You tell yourself that it is what it is. You see that you are not your problem. You think about what you do want. You stay focused on what you want and acknowledge every small win. You make peace with where you are and keep creating with your focus.

When you can get this to become your habitual thought process, you will stop identifying with things in your life and see yourself as you truly are--a powerful creator. Your self-image will be built from whatever you want it to be, and you will be confident that you can have whatever you want in your life.

"Live your truth. Express your love. Share your enthusiasm.
Take action towards your dreams. Walk your talk.
Dance and sing to your music. Embrace your blessings.
Make today worth remembering."

Dr Steve Maraboli

Chapter 10

Rolling with the Punches

I OFTEN GET asked if I ever have a bad day. The short answer is NO. I say this because for me, having a bad day is a decision. I may have a bad moment that lasts an hour or so but making a day of it does not light me up. So I decide to have a good day, and I focus on things that bring me joy.

The long answer is still no. I have had no shortage of very challenging times in my life, some that have taken all my energy and focus to overcome or even survive. Things happen that activate fear and doubt in me, but I am very careful that I never let it take hold. I know that it is a very slippery slope that can leave me paralyzed by fear before I know what hit me. My thoughts and focus are priceless to me, and I will never let an external situation or circumstance control them. I made a commitment to myself to be normal and happy when I was a teenager, and I have never broken it. I learned to control my thoughts and focus so that no matter what was going on around me, I would have a good day.

Sound like a pipe dream? It didn't happen overnight. It took practice to be able to control my thoughts and choose my emotional state. I wasn't very good when I first started. My heart was rarely behaving the way I wanted, and kids were always being mean to me. Not only would I be upset and have a bad day but I'd also beat myself up because I could not ignore these things and focus on the good.

Fortunately, I learned that thinking about things I liked and distracting myself could stop my crying faster than consolation from someone well-meaning. Adults were telling me that no one should treat me that way and that it is so unfair that this has happened to me. This just made me feel worse. I got much better results by forgetting about it, feeling good and never looking back.

Once I found out how well this strategy worked, I applied it to everything. Being in a bad mood made any situation much worse than it was. In fact, I rarely, if ever, solved any problems when I was in a bad mood. When I made being in a good mood my priority, it was almost like I stopped having problems because I got so good at solving them.

I didn't avoid what was going on in my life. I just avoided the things I did not like for long enough to get happy. Once I was in a good mood, I saw the situation through different eyes, and somehow things seemed okay. This is the reason why I am committed to never having a bad day ever again. The cost is far too high, and my happiness is the most important thing in the world to me.

I know that there will always be changes happening in my life. Maybe they will be related to my condition, my business, my family or my personal life. I don't know what will happen and I know that it is futile to spend time worrying about things I don't want and worst case scenarios. My goal is to be happy and normal. In order to make that the case, no matter what happens around me, my job is to roll with the punches daily and find something to appreciate in my life and make it my dominant focus.

I have been doing this all my life, and it has worked to build me a wonderful life full of everything I could ask for. Life gives me opportunities. It does not impose limitations on me. Even if circumstances seem to make it impossible for me to do or achieve something in the moment, I remind myself that I have just not seen the path yet. If I want it badly enough, and I keep my thoughts positive and my focus on what I want, it will happen.

This is the way life is supposed to work. I know this through applying it and living it. Now, in my study of personal growth, mindset and the law of attraction, I have found plenty of experts and books who back up what I'm telling you. They all just seem to keep validating what I have already known. It's a wonderful way to live, and there is no reason why everyone can't do it. Sadly, most people don't, but if you've read until this point, I know that you want to.

When you have a heart condition, there are definitely more variables to consider in your day to day life. They can and will grab at your focus, and the tendency is to let them lead you down that slippery slope. Here is my strategy for staying the course and making sure that I always have a good day.

Always Make Sure that Your Dominant Focus is on What You Want

See the life that you want to be living clearly in your mind. Visualize yourself living and doing the activities that you will be doing when you get what you want. You want to see it so clearly in your mind that you actually get the emotional feeling that you would have if it were physically happening. You create it and live the experience in your mind first and then it happens in your life physically.

I can hardly even count how many open heart surgeries I have had in my life. Back in 2008, it was really hard on me because I had four surgeries back to back within months. I know full well that any surgery can be life-threatening and when I think that way I get scared. That activates the fear and doubt so I never even go there because it makes the experience bad for me and everyone involved. Instead, I visualize myself already done the surgery and everyone I love sitting around me being happy. I see myself as healthy and enjoying the positive results that the successful procedure has created in my life.

Stuff Isn't Good or Bad Until You Decide It Is

Stuff Happens. Things will change. Life goes on. Nothing has any meaning until you decide that it does. You choose the meaning and life unfolds accordingly. The secret is not to jump to any conclusions. Don't let your mind automatically tell you that something is bad, just because you have always reacted that way.

It's okay to catch yourself reacting and labeling a situation as bad. Just stop and look at the circumstances for what they are, without any judgment. Tell yourself that this event is neutral. It means nothing about me or my life. Trust me. Doing this opens up a world of possibility. Jumping to a negative conclusion only gives you one bad one.

As I am writing this book, my doctors are still trying to figure out why my device has been shocking me and what to do about it. I've only just been given the go-ahead to ease back into the physical activity regime that delights and energizes me so much. Many times, my thoughts and emotions were starting to head down that negative path. I'd be thinking, "Here we go again" but before that turned into a whole vivid scene of my life being over, I'd switch my thought. I'd think about how grateful I was for technology that has allowed me to live such a rich and full life. I'd thank God that I live in a time where there are solutions for me to keep living well. If I had been born even ten years earlier, there might not have been options to keep me alive.

Decide How You Want Things to Be

I know that everything in my life always works out. In the moment, I may not be getting what I expected, but I trust the grand scheme of things. I tell myself in the moment that this is on the path to what I want. Then I go back to focusing on what I want.

When the circumstances in your life are not exactly the way you want them to be, you have to let that go. That situation has already been created by past reactions, judgments, thoughts, feelings, and focus. Make peace with yourself and know that in this moment you can decide how you want things to be. You get to create a new reality in every moment, and now you are serious. Get a clear picture in your mind of what you want and decide that it is going to happen.

My specialist has been talking about another surgery to try to correct what is going on with my device and the neurons in my heart. I have decided that I want to create a new neural pathway in my heart that works better than it did before. I keep visualizing this pathway, and I see myself participating in all the activities I want to do with energy and vigour. I don't know how the result will be delivered to me, but I do know that I will be back at my high-intensity workouts with my heart supporting me all the way.

Do What You Need to Do to Get Happy

Whenever we want something that we don't have, inevitably, it's because we think we'll feel better or be happier by having it. The real end result that we are looking for is to feel good and be happy. We may think that we are not happy because we don't have what we want but the fact of the matter is that we are not being happy. Being happy and having what you want are two different things. It's possible to have what you want and not be happy, and you can also be happy without having what you want.

The big secret to attracting what you want into your life is knowing how to be happy even though you don't have what you want. Being happy puts you in an attractive state, and things start working out for you. When you are happy, problems melt away, and the possibilities seem to multiply.

The big problem most people face is that they can't think about the thing they want in their life without feeling a negative emotion about the fact that it's not there. As long as you experience negative emotions when you think about the thing you want, you are more in alignment with the lack of it, and you aren't going to attract it. When you can think about it with excitement, and you can see yourself experiencing it clearly in your mind, what you want will soon be yours.

Doing whatever you need to do to be happy is the fastest way to get everything you want. Even when things are not going your way, find something to think about that makes you happy. Watch a funny movie or read something inspiring. Laugh your butt off at crazy animal videos. Make happiness and feeling good your number one priority and you will be well on your way to whatever you want.

Take Inspired Action

I'm all about taking small actions that add up to big results, but your state of mind when you act is the key. There is a big difference between doing something because you know you should do it and taking action because you want to. By focusing on what you want and making sure that you are happy, you will find yourself inspired into action. There is nothing more powerful than inspired action.

If you feel grudgingly about something that you are about to do, don't do it. Exercising and eating a healthy diet because your doctor said you had to is not going to be very effective. When you are inspired to exercise and excited about making nutritional choices that will fuel your body, the very same actions that your doctor recommended all of a sudden become 100 times more powerful.

Exercising and eating healthy have always been a passion of mine. No one ever has to tell me to exercise, and I am always looking for ways to care for my body even better with good nutrition. As a result, I feel empowered when I take these actions, and the results in my body are phenomenal.

When I drag my butt to the gym because I feel guilty, those are the days that something goes wrong or I don't get the results I want.

I know that not everyone has the same motivations as I do. Not everyone will want to do wind sprints and lift heavy weight. I started by simply wanting to do some cardio. I knew I had some limitations to work with because of my device so I asked my doctor how I should go about getting active. As I got more into it, I was asking more questions and doing more research to find ways that I could do the things that I wanted to do. Whenever I had a new challenge, a new question would pop into my mind, and new answers started to come my way. I am forever googling the questions I have about my heart.

Everything Happens for a Reason but It's up to You to Find Yours

If everything that happens in life is neutral and nothing has any meaning until you assign your own meaning to it, then you get to decide what life means. Everyone is already deciding their meaning of life, and most people have chosen a pretty sad one. They say they don't know what it is or why things happen because they are expecting some grand revelation. Meanwhile, they go on doing the same thing every day and complaining about how bad things are. They let others tell them what things mean which is really dangerous because they get sucked into the negative social perspective. But it doesn't have to be this way!

You just need to decide that from now on, you decide what the meaning is. If other people don't agree, just ignore them. Their meaning is more than likely going to be rather dismal. It's up to you to decide what you want things to mean and then surround yourself with people that buy into your reality. If you have decided to be happy at all costs, think of how happy all the people around you are going to have to be! Yes, some of your friends may not be very happy with you for trying to be happy all the time. You may have to let some people in your life go and develop some radically new ways of dealing with the people who you can't get away from.

Most of all you need to find a cheerleader. For me, that person is my husband. Back in 2008 when I had had three open heart surgeries and was scheduled for a fourth, I was really struggling with the toll it was taking on me. I told him that I did not think I could make it through another surgery. Our daughter, who was 12 years old at the time and has always been very headstrong. He said, "Wait just a minute. You're not leaving me to raise her all by myself!" I said, "You're right! You would totally screw her up!" Then we both laughed, and I made it through. I could not have done it without him.

My son thinks that having this heart condition is somehow related to my purpose in life. I agree. I wasn't born with it, and I was healthy and athletic right up until I was 12. They never could find a cause other than hypothesizing that maybe a virus had attacked my heart. Maybe I can put a new face on this condition. People are so used to hearing so much negativity around it. I'm just grateful for every experience I have had because of this condition and the beautiful life I have created from all I have learned in living with it.

How about you? Maybe your condition is more complex

or life-threatening. Maybe it's not. I never compare myself to other people because you will never win at that game. Too many people make their lives all about how sick they are, and it is the only way they know how to relate to others. I could have been the sick and frail little girl my whole life, but I probably would be dead by now. I would rather just roll with the punches and keep on living to see what other marvelous adventures life has to reveal to me.

Contact Linda at
lmwn51@yahoo.ca

CPSIA information can be obtained
at www.ICGtesting.com
Printed in the USA
LVHW05s2231011018
592068LV00002B/3/P